A DOCTOR'S
PERSPECTIVE ON
CBD

Green & Natural Publishing
(Green & Natural Publishing is a wholly-owned subsidiary of IN8Wellness LLC)
54541 Hunter's Ct
Elkhart, IN 46514

ISBN: 978-1-7337944-0-4 (print)
ISBN: 978-1-7337944-1-1 (ebook)

Ordering Information:

Special discounts are available on quantity purchases by corporations, associations, and others. For details, contact Green & Natural Publishing via email: IN8Wellnessllc@gmail.com.

A DOCTOR'S PERSPECTIVE ON

CBD

Science, Success Stories, and Changed Lives

DR. MARK LINDHOLM
CHIROPRACTOR

Health Disclaimer

CONTENTS

FIRST THOUGHTS FROM THE CLINIC

You or someone you love is likely suffering with health problems. You hope and pray that something will change.

You've heard that CBD oil may help, but you worry about the connection to marijuana. Is it safe? Will you get high? Can I pass a drug test? Will I become a stoner? Is it snake oil? Whose lives have been changed by CBD?

I have worked with hundreds of patients who arrived with those exact worries. Using CBD, these same people have gotten dramatic relief from chronic pain, anxiety, depression, problems sleeping, and PTSD. Many reported improved focus and concentration. One became seizure free from using only CBD and is able to drive and work again. Others with digestive problems, diabetes, infections, and swelling all report improvement with CBD that was unlike anything they had previously experienced. A young woman I know had a brain tumor and believes CBD saved her life.

The science, research, and studies inside will back up what I've seen with my own eyes and give you a grasp on the possibilities of CBD and the endocannabinoid system, even if you're brand new to this topic.

In addition, there are personal testimonials where people like you will describe how their lives have changed, even my own painful story, which sent me on a journey to discover what type of CBD is best so I could help others recover.

I pray that each of you learn and benefit from the information contained in the pages of this book. I hope you'll be inspired to take action and improve your health and the health of those you love.

CHAPTER TWO

TURNING PAIN INTO A NEW LIFE

I was scared my 25-year career as a chiropractor was over.

The plan was for me to move a Japanese maple tree from the front of my new clinic to my yard at home. I grabbed a shovel and started digging, but as I dug the roots seemed to go everywhere and I reached a point when the tree just wouldn't budge. I vigorously began to attack the roots, and one of my thrusts sent excruciating pain through my right wrist. I immediately knew it wasn't a small problem. I tried to fight through it and returned to work, but the pain didn't go away. It got worse.

You can't adjust someone's spine without using your wrist. All day long, you're pushing, twisting, and putting tremendous force on your wrist. Every single adjustment I made on a patient caused me pain that, over time, started to travel up my arm and into my shoulder and neck. My muscles tightened because the nerves were irritated.

I struggled through work for weeks, and I had to drink three or four glasses of wine to deaden the ache when I returned home. Then I went right to bed because I knew I had to get up and do it all over again in the morning. The pain prevented me from doing much of anything else. Just as difficult as dealing with the physical pain was the emotional stress as time went on and my condition worsened.

Adjusting the spine is an art form. It's like learning how to play the violin or the piano. It's not something everyone can do, and it took me well over 25 years to hone my skills as a chiropractor. A long-term wrist injury could easily diminish my skills and turn me into a second-rate chiropractor or, even worse, force me to retire. I love to interact with my patients and witness the miracles that can occur with the kind of care we give them. It's not just about providing for my family—working as a chiropractor is my passion, and it's what drives me in life. I love to go to work every day. I don't know what else I'd do.

I've wanted to be a chiropractor since I was a little kid. It started when I was five years old and suffered from extreme stomach pains that became so severe I spent most of my days sick in bed. My parents took me to see multiple doctors but they never found anything wrong with me. Even the specialists couldn't give my parents any concrete answers. One of my father's coworkers recommended a chiropractor named, Dr. Nelson, but my parents had never been to one. They assumed that a chiropractor only dealt with back problems so they didn't see how she could possibly help with my chronic stomach pain.

One day after I received another battery of tests at the hospital, my parents drove past Dr. Nelson's office. Frustrated by the situation and by the fact that I wasn't getting any better, they decided to stop. As luck would have it, the doctor could fit us in. She examined my spine and explained to my parents that I had some subluxations in the middle of my thoracic spine that could be irritating the nerves.

I was only five years old so I don't remember much about that day in detail, but I do remember that after she performed that first adjustment, I felt instant relief. The next day, my stomach pain was 70-80 percent better. My parents noticed so much of a change that when the hospital called back to say that the latest round of tests revealed I had an ulcer, my mom told the doctors that we were going to wait and see how I responded to the chiropractic treatment before exploring further medical options.

I went back to Dr. Nelson for more adjustments, and after only a month, the pain and the problem were gone entirely. Dr. Nelson explained to us how the problem wasn't really in my stomach. It was coming from the nerves that controlled my stomach. Half of the nerves that control the stomach come from the thoracic spine. She couldn't prove it, but the chiropractor theorized that the pressure on the nerves made the stomach secrete too much acid, causing the ulcer. The adjustments corrected the problem instead of covering up the symptoms. I don't know this for sure but there is a chance that if I returned to the hospital and underwent treatment, it could have left that subluxation irritating the nerves and the problem would never have been corrected.

Nobody ever needed to tell me about the benefit of seeing a chiropractor because I experienced it at such a young age. Now that I've been a practicing chiropractor for 25 years, I see miraculous results all the time. I consider it a blessing. I get to work with God's wonderful creation—the human body—and all I'm doing is removing any interference so nerves can work the way they are intended. My job is my passion, which was why I was so devastated when it looked like it was going to be taken away from me.

For weeks after my wrist injury, I saw multiple doctors and tried everything that helped my patients with similar ailments. I got regular adjustments. I took nutritional supplements and got massages. I even had a colleague do laser treatments on my wrist. None of it helped so I started taking antiinflammatory medication, which is something as a chiropractor that I have not done in decades. It didn't help much, either.

I had recently heard about hemp-derived CBD oil, which was legal in my home state of Indiana. If you had asked me a year earlier if CBD would help to alleviate the type of severe pain I experienced in my wrist, I would have said no way. Once I learned how hemp was different from marijuana, I felt like I didn't have anything to lose so I tried it.

I didn't expect it to work but I felt the pain in my wrist lessen within days. Work became more tolerable. The longer I used CBD oil, the more profound the benefits became and my wrist eventually healed. It saved my career and allowed me to continue working.

I believe things happen for a reason and that there are no real coincidences in this world. About two months later, I attended a chiropractic conference in California. I looked forward to that conference every year, not just because sunny California provided a nice respite from the cold and dreary weather in Indiana, but because it was one of the most amazing conferences in the chiropractic world.

That year, three of the keynote speakers talked about the health benefits of hemp-derived CBD oil and how it showed results with pain, anxiety, cancer, and immune function while being completely safe. I was blown away by what the experts said and immediately looked into making the product available to my patients. I was so excited when I returned home to Indiana that I researched and read everything I could get my hands on. I spent months reading journals, reviewing PubMed studies online, watching videos and webinars, and looking at CBD companies to find the very best product.

After spending countless hours studying and trying products myself, I thought I knew all about CBD. It wasn't until I introduced the product to my patients and saw their results first-hand that my education really began.

CHAPTER THREE

HEMP, CBD, & MARIJUANA: WHAT'S THE DIFFERENCE?

CBD was undoubtedly popular but not all of my patients were open to it because they didn't understand it. Many felt that it was the equivalent of marijuana, which they didn't want other people to think they were using. Others asked about CBD precisely because they thought it had the same effect as marijuana.

Put simply, the hemp plant is a cousin to the marijuana plant. It's similar to the difference between sweet corn and field corn. Hemp is the parent plant, and cannabis is the scientific name for that plant. Both hemp and marijuana contain cannabidiol, or CBD. As recreational marijuana use became more popular, the marijuana plant was hybridized to produce more than 40 times the amount of THC, the chemical responsible for marijuana's psychological or "high" effects. Hemp, on the other hand, has a very low amount of THC. In fact, for a CBD product to be legal, it must have less than 0.3% THC, and the product must also be a hemp-derived CBD.

Not only does hemp have a very low amount of THC compared to marijuana but it also has more significant health benefits when compared with THC or any of the other 100-plus compounds (cannabinoids) that have been isolated in the cannabis plant. A study published in the *Journal of Pharmacology and Experimental Therapeutics*[1] investigated the anti-tumor activities of five different cannabinoids. Of the five natural compounds tested, CBD was the most potent inhibitor of cancer cell growth.

The study suggests that you don't need THC because the CBD portion is the most potent and effective component. That means you benefit from using the non-psychoactive (and perfectly legal) CBD portion without what some consider the detrimental effects of THC. This is important, especially for individuals who can't or don't want to risk testing positive for marijuana.

THE LEGALITY OF IT ALL

Many people continue to lump CBD and THC together because they are both considered cannabis and, for a long time, they were illegal. The legal issues with hemp can be

---

1 Ligresti A, Moriello AS, Starowicz K, Matias I, Pisanti S, De Petrocellis L, Laezza C, Portella G, Bifulco M, Di Marzo V. "Antitumor activity of plant cannabinoids with emphasis on the effect of cannabidiol on human breast carcinoma." *The Journal of Pharmacology and Experimental Therapeutics*. 2006, September; 318(3): 1375-87. EPUB 2006 May 25.

traced back to the Marihuana Tax Act of 1937 that placed a tax on the sale of cannabis. This tax act had nothing to do with hemp being dangerous and everything to do with business and politics.

Hemp was used for making paper and clothing. Some of the influential businessmen of the time were scared of competition from the hemp industry and set out to eliminate that competition by making it illegal. Additionally, racist, anti-Mexican sentiment contributed to the villainization of hemp. To accomplish their goal, they created the term marijuana (or "marihuana," as it was called at the time) to define all hemp and cannabis products.

Some believe that the creation of the word marijuana was an attempt not just to malign the use of hemp but also to disguise the real intention of the act. Had it been called The Hemp Tax Act, it might not have passed. Even the American Medical Association opposed the act because hemp was such a valuable commodity and was widely prescribed by doctors and pharmacists at that time.

THE HISTORY OF HEMP

Hemp is one of the oldest cultivated crops in human history. It has been used in medicine and to make goods such as clothing, rope, sails, and paper. Archaeologists have discovered cloth made from hemp in Mesopotamia that dates back 10,000 years while ancient Chinese writings document the herbal and medicinal use of hemp seeds and oils. In ancient Rome, Nero's army surgeon included hemp in his medical inventory.

Even in the United States, there is a long history of hemp. Early Jamestown settlers observed Powhatan Indians growing hemp in 1607. Years later, colonial farmers could be fined by the British government if they did not grow hemp, whose fibers were used to make rope and sails for the British Navy. Early drafts of the Declaration of Independence were written on hemp paper. Later, pharmaceutical companies became one of the largest users of hemp and hemp oil[2].

"Cannabis has been used to treat pain for thousands of years. However, since the early part of the twentieth century, laws restricting cannabis use have limited its evaluation using modern scientific criteria," concluded a September 2017 study in Clinical and Experimental Rheumatology[3]. "Over the last decade, the situation has started to change because of the increased availability of cannabis in the United States for either medical or recreational purposes, making it important to provide the public with accurate information as to the effectiveness of the drug for joint pain among other indications."

The truth is that hemp is not a drug. It's a plant that provides phytocannabinoids, which naturally enhance the human body's endocannabinoid system (ECS). The ECS is a biological system with receptors for these naturally made or

2   "A Hemp History Lesson," Zilis.com/drmark and *Colonial Williamsburg Journal: Winter 2015*: "Hemp & Flax in Colonial America," History.org.
3   Miller RJ, Miller RE, "Is cannabis an effective treatment for joint pain?" *Clinical and Experimental Rheumatology*, 2017 Sep-Oct: 35 Suppl 107 (5): 59-67. EPUB 2017 Sept 28.

endogenous cannabinoids found throughout the body. We even have receptors for these health-promoting chemicals in our circulating white blood cells.

You can think of the ECS like a hormonal system. Any woman will tell you that her hormones affect not just her monthly menstruation cycles but also how she feels all over, from her mood and skin complexion to her energy levels and digestion. In a similar way, the ECS affects the entire body and is the major contributor to balance in the body for a vertebrate (humans and any animal with a backbone). The phytocannabinoids in the hemp plant interact with these same receptors to help enhance the ECS.

We are still learning about the ECS, but what is clear is that it impacts the entire body, including the cardiovascular system (heart and circulation), digestive system (stomach and intestines), endocrine system (hormones), exocrine system (liver, pancreas, breast milk, sweat, saliva, and mucus), musculoskeletal system (bones and muscles), immune system (fights against infection and abnormal or cancerous cells), renal system (kidneys involved in elimination of waste, control of blood chemical levels, and blood pressure), nervous system (the master controller of your body), reproductive system (sexual function and the miracle of new life), and the respiratory system (breathing, removal of carbon dioxide, and taking in of oxygen)[4].

4 Natalia Battista, Monia Di Tommaso, Monica Bari, and Mauro Maccarrone, "The Endocannabinoid system an overview, Frontiers in Behavioral Neuroscience," Published online 2012 Mar 14.

WHY I RECOMMEND CBD TO MY PATIENTS

CBD is a supplement that appealed to me because it's enormously effective for so many health issues like anxiety, heart disease, acne, sleeping problems, pain and inflammation, cancer, diabetes, and seizures, and CBD comes from a natural plant. That's important to me because I believe in a nonsurgical and drug-free approach to healthcare whenever possible. It's the root of what I do as a chiropractor. I don't prescribe drugs or perform surgery, and I believe patients should seek natural remedies first, drugs as a second approach, and surgery as a last resort.

I often collaborate with other doctors in my community to help patients, and sometimes medication is necessary. But the general public is starting to understand that every drug has side effects so the fewer drugs you can take, the better off you are. I'm always trying to decrease my patients' dependency on drugs, and often that means working with their medical physician to reduce their dosage or eventually discontinue certain medications altogether. It's important that you always seek the advice of your doctor and healthcare provider to discuss all of the treatment options available to you, and I've always felt it is worth exploring other avenues.

Very few people know about CBD studies, and patients ask me all the time why they haven't heard about it being used to treat various conditions. The fact is, high-quality medical literature is available on the benefits of CBD that anyone can access but it can be difficult for the layperson to understand. PubMed, for instance, is an online repository of medical and scientific studies managed and supported by the National Institutes of Health. However, reading these studies is almost like deciphering another language if you don't understand the medical terminology or know what to look for. For that reason, I will break down these studies and explain the research in a way that's easy for everyone to understand because some of the findings are truly remarkable.

I've been using and recommending supplements to my patients for more than two decades, and I've seen some incredible results, but nothing compared to the astounding results I began to see from my patients after they started taking CBD. It was life-changing for many of them. Some noticed results after taking the product only for a week but most patients experienced the maximum benefit when they used the product every day for two or three months. I'd often recommend the product to patients for one problem, and not only would that ailment improve but they also would notice other improvements in their overall health. In other words, they experienced side benefits instead of side effects.

Why does this product have such profound effects on our overall health? It's because we all have the endocannabinoid system in our bodies, even if it wasn't discovered until the 1990s. Many experts say our body is designed to use these phytocannabinoids or plant-based cannabinoids via our endocannabinoid system or natural innate cannabinoid system. We have receptors throughout our bodies to which these plant-based and self-made or endogenous canna-binoids "bind." When this happens, it causes a balancing effect or homeostasis that promotes health, but a deficiency in the body's natural endocannabinoids exists in modern times perhaps because hemp has been considered an illegal substance for more than 80 years[5].

Before the 1937 Marijuana Tax Act, hemp was used for medicinal purposes. It was also widely fed to animals and sometimes eaten directly by people. It was ubiquitous, and people received benefits by merely eating products from animals that were fed hemp or hemp seeds. When hemp was made illegal, people no longer got phytocannabinoids in their diet.

Imagine if you took a staple product, such as eggs, and re-moved it from the average American diet overnight. That's what happened with hemp. Once regulations were enacted, the only hemp that could be used had to be imported because it wasn't legal to grow the plant in the United States. It couldn't even be studied at universities since it was grouped with all cannabis species as a Schedule I drug in the Controlled Substance Act of 1970. That's the same classification as a drug like cocaine.

---

5   "Health benefits of hemp seeds," Tue 11 September 2018 By Cathleen Crichton-Stuart, *Health News Today.*

THE CHANGING LANDSCAPE

Fast forward to 2014, when the United States government passed a new pilot program through the Farm Bill that would allow hemp to be grown and studied. Individual states have expanded on that by making hemp and marijuana legal to use medicinally and recreationally.

Every four years, the Farm Bill has to be reapproved, but permanent language in the Hemp Farming Act of 2018, which falls under the Farm Bill, changed the status of hemp from a Controlled I substance to a commodity like corn, soybeans, or tobacco.

This bill has far-reaching implications for the hemp industry, American farmers, and the nation's economy. It should dispel much of the confusion between marijuana and hemp and greatly reduce regulations while resulting in an explosion of the industry. The change not only significantly promises to improve the medicinal market but it also may lead to hemp potentially becoming a huge cash crop for US farmers, replacing millions of dollars of imported hemp. Many authorities predict that the hemp industry could grow a minimum of 700 percent[6]. Some experts forecast that soon hemp will be planted in the Midwest as much as corn.

I predict that most Americans within the next five years will

---

6 Debra Borchardt, "The Cannabis Market That Could Grow 700% By 2020," *Forbes*, Dec 12, 2016 and Grace Dobush, "Why the U.S. Cannabis Industry May Witness a $20 Billion Boom," *Fortune*, December 13, 2018.

have at least tried a CBD product and a high percentage will use it on a regular basis like they now use multivitamins or other supplements to promote health. (Read "A Personal Note from the Author" at the end of this book and go to www.CBDdrmark.com if you want more information about the financial opportunities of getting involved at the ground floor level in this dramatically growing CBD and Hemp industry.)

CHAPTER FOUR

HOW SAFE IS CBD?

Safety is an extremely important issue. When I advise my patients about any treatment or supplement, the first thing I consider is its safety, and the second thing is its effectiveness.

Study after study in this book shows how effective CBD is in treating conditions such as epilepsy, pain, arthritis, inflammation of the joints and digestive system, autoimmune disorders as well as maintaining healthy blood sugar levels, regulating the immune system, and even helping to kill cancer cells. I've witnessed the effectiveness of CBD in the patients in my clinic. There is definitely more research to be done, but the science backs it up and is clearly documented in this book so let's cross effectiveness off the list.

Now, what about the safety of CBD? (When I reference CBD, I'm referring to a full-spectrum hemp oil CBD like the product I sell at my clinic.)

A June 2017 literature review[7] looked at 74 total studies on the safety of CBD and found promising results.

"In general, the often-described favorable safety profile of CBD in humans was confirmed and extended by the reviewed research," the review said.

Most of the studies looked at the treatment of epilepsy and psychotic disorders. The most common side effects were drowsiness, diarrhea, and changes in appetite and weight. Compared to other drugs, CBD has fewer side effects, which may be why patients might be more likely to use CBD and follow through with treatment, according to the review. It went on to say more clinical research is warranted, but that CBD had the potential to reduce the need for other drugs in patients with epilepsy.

Are natural products like CBD 100 percent safe? Can we say that nobody will have an adverse reaction to it? Absolutely not. We can't say that about anything because people can have all kinds of allergic and negative responses to all types of products. However, study after study confirms that CBD is well tolerated and has an excellent safety profile, especially when compared to the pharmaceutical drugs regularly used to treat these serious conditions.

7   Iffland, Kerstin., Grotenhermen, Franjo., "An Update on Safety and Side Effects of Cannabidiol: A Review of Clinical Data and Relevant Animal Studies," *Cannabis and Cannabinoid Research*, 2017; 2(1): 139-154. Published online 2017 June 1.

CAN I GET ADDICTED?

The first question I get from the more skeptical patients to whom I recommend CBD is, "Isn't that just pot?" The second question I typically get is, "Can I get addicted?"

We've already established that CBD is not the same as marijuana, and for a CBD oil to be sold legally in the United States, it has to contain less than 0.3 percent THC. I would suggest, however, that you find a product like the one I use in my clinic that has zero percent THC.

When taking a pure CBD product, you don't risk being exposed to any of the potentially addictive or harmful components of THC. As important, you also don't have to worry about testing positive for marijuana. You could test positive if you take other CBD or hemp products out on the market today, even if they are at or slightly under the 0.3% legal limit.

In November 2017, the World Health Organization published its report on CBD at a meeting held by their Expert Committee on Drug Dependence.[8] It claimed there have been no reported cases of physical dependence or withdrawal from CBD, nor any reported cases of abuse or public health problems related to the use of CBD.

Many of the studies throughout the book mention the need for further research and that is most definitely true but it

8   World Health Organization, Expert Committee on Drug Dependence, "Cannabidiol (CBD) Pre-Review Report, Agenda Item 5.2., Thirty-ninth Meeting, Geneva, 6-10, November 2017.

shouldn't cause any concerns about potential safety issues. I often tell my patients that new drugs aren't the safest drugs on the market (even if they have received FDA approval) because they haven't survived the test of time.

Hemp, however, has passed the test of time. Some of the earliest written evidence of hemp's medicinal use comes from ancient China, where it was administered to the emperor in 2737 B.C. Fast forward thousands of years to 77 A.D., when there is written evidence of the Romans using hemp for medicinal purposes. Hemp was popular in the Middle East and in India, where it was considered a sacred grass and used for centuries as medicine. This history doesn't just go back one or two generations but for thousands of years, which (along with contemporary research) adds to hemp's reputation for safety.

IS IT POSSIBLE TO OVERDOSE?

While CBD is absorbed by the body, it's unlikely you'll overdose.

Current Drug Safety published a report[9] that proved CBD to be nontoxic. Even high doses up to 1500 milligrams per day—90 times the amount I recommend to my patients on a daily basis—were well tolerated in humans. The dose I recommend for my patients is only 16 milligrams per day, and it's been getting amazing results.

9   Bergamaschi MM., Queiroz RH., Zuardi AW., Crippa JA., "Safety and side effects of cannabidiol, a Cannabis sativa constituent," *Current Drug Safety,* 2011 Sept 1;6(4): 237-49.

"Based on recent advances in cannabinoid administration in humans, controlled CBD may be safe in humans and animals," the report concluded.

CBD AND OTHER MEDICATIONS

The Journal of Addiction Medicine[10] also published a study that looked at the safety of CBD when used by patients being treated for opioid addiction with fentanyl.

This was a double-blind, placebo-controlled crossover study conducted at Mount Sinai Hospital in New York City, which by any measure makes it a quality study. Researchers looked specifically to see if it was safe to use CBD while taking drugs for opioid addiction and the results were positive: "These data provide the foundation for future studies examining CBD as a potential treatment for opioid abuse."

There is some indication that blood pressure medications might be more effective, meaning that patients might be able to use a lower dose of their blood pressure medication when taking a CBD product. Similarly, if someone is taking a blood pressure medication, they might want to start out more slowly with CBD because it could cause an excessive drop in blood pressure. In addition to consulting with their medical physician, I recommend that patients not take the

10 Alex F. Manini, Georgia Yiannoulos, Mateus M. Bergamaschi, Stephanie Hernandez ,Ruben Olmedo, Allan J. Barnes, Gary Winkel, Rajita Sinha, Didier Jutras-Aswad, Marilyn A. Huestis, Yasmin L. Hurd, "Safety and pharmacokinetics of oral cannabidiol when administered concomitantly with intravenous fentanyl in humans," *The Journal of Addiction Medicine,* 2015 May-Jun; 9(3): 204-210.

two medications at the same time until they know how their body will react.

CHAPTER FIVE

HOW MUCH DO I TAKE?

Everyone is different. Factors such as your weight and height, diet, metabolism, genetics, environment, and life-style all could potentially affect your optimal CBD dose. Because there is no universal dose, it's important to point out that the information in this chapter is intended to serve only as a guide. It's a starting point and should not be considered medical advice.

Many of the best full-spectrum hemp oil CBD products on the market come in a bottle with a dropper that you use to administer the liquid under your tongue. I tell my patients to shake the bottle and use about half a dropper of the product—or about 8 milligrams per dose. Hold it there for about a minute before swallowing. I tell most of them to do this twice a day for 16 milligrams total per day.

The idea is to separate each dose by about 12 hours (usually at morning and at night) to achieve a 24-hour saturation in the body of therapeutic levels of CBD. This is the dose I recommend, but patients respond differently. Some do well with half of what I recommend, while others require higher doses.

I've been a chiropractor long enough to know that people don't always do exactly what I recommend. For instance, when one of my patients said that she hadn't noticed anything different after using the product for a couple of weeks, I had to make sure that she was using it correctly.

"Have you been using it every day?" I asked.

"Yeah, I think I only missed one day," she said.

"Have you been putting it under your tongue?"

"Yes."

"How much of it have you been taking?" I asked.

"Well, that's the funny thing. You told me to take half a drop twice a day, but how do you get half a drop out of the dropper?"

I couldn't help but explode with laughter. "Nancy," I said, "you're supposed to take half a dropper full, not half a drop."

Lo and behold, after she started using the product as intended, she got results.

ABSORPTION IS THE KEY

The fact that there are so many different CBD products, and they are absorbed by the body at different rates, makes this even more complicated. Absorption can be drastically different from one product to the next, making it difficult to establish a standard dose.

Oil and water don't mix, and since the human body is primarily water, CBD oil isn't naturally absorbed. Most CBD products on the market have an absorbability level of three to six percent. Absorption also can be delayed because oils and fats need to travel through the digestive system and then be broken down to be effectively absorbed into the body.

In my personal practice, I've witnessed great results by having patients use a water-soluble product absorbed at 80-94 percent. About 20 milligrams of a regular CBD oil with only 3-6 percent absorption will have a very different effect than the same amount of a product that is water soluble and is 80-94 percent absorbed.

It's not what you swallow that matters—it's what's getting absorbed!

THERE ARE ALWAYS EXCEPTIONS

I have a friend with a very severe chronic injury who had been taking opioids for 14 years. He needed a much higher dose of CBD than the average person. He told me that during those 14 years, he went through detox twice, which involved being curled up in the fetal position, vomiting, and suffering with diarrhea for two days.

"Detox is not pleasant!" he told me.

When he used the product from my clinic, he got amazing results and was able to get off of his opioids without the usual detox issues. Now, when he starts to feel the panic and anxiety of opioid withdrawal, he takes a second dropper full of CBD oil and those feelings are gone in 10 to 15 minutes. CBD helped free him from opioid dependence.

I also have patients with chronic pain and inflammation who require a higher dose. It's good to know that there is no level of CBD that is considered hazardous, and even chronic high-use doses up to 1500 milligrams per day have been repeatedly shown to be well tolerated in humans.

I have other patients with more chronic problems such as degenerative arthritis, bone-on-bone arthritis in their knee, or severe arthritis in their spine who don't experience dramatic results from CBD because it can't regrow cartilage or cause the discs in the spine to regenerate. The mechanical problem will still be there, no matter how much CBD they take.

However, many of these patients have found that the product helped them more than they expected. Several patients have told me things like, "You know, I wasn't really sure that the CBD oil I got from you was helping, but I ran out of it two weeks ago and couldn't wait to get back in and get some more because my pain returned."

It's also difficult to come up with a universal dose standard because the way people respond to CBD can vary dramatically. I've had patients say they noticed an improvement relatively quickly. This appears to happen more in people suffering from depression, anxiety, or sleep problems. They often notice a difference within a week or sometimes even after a single dose. Whether or not someone experiences early benefits, I try to make it clear that it can take up to a month or two to really get the full benefit of the product.

With all of that in mind, I recommend that people find a full-spectrum hemp oil CBD product that is water soluble and start by taking 15 to 20 milligrams a day, split between two doses. Remember, it's okay to start with a small dose and gradually increase if needed.

CHAPTER SIX

QUESTIONS TO ASK ABOUT CBD PRODUCTS

We've already proven that CBD is safe and effective, but there are six criteria to keep in mind when deciding which product you should purchase.

1) IS IT ORGANIC?

You want a product that is USDA Certified Organic. This is even more important with hemp than it is for organic fruits and vegetables. Hemp is an extremely efficient plant at taking up nutrients, which is part of the reason for its nickname "weed." It absorbs vitamins and minerals but also can absorb impurities like pesticides, herbicides, and heavy metals. It literally cleans the ground, so if you aren't buying organic hemp, there is a chance you're getting those toxins and chemicals in your CBD.

2) HOW IS IT PROCESSED?

You want to look for a product that is processed in a natural way using CO2 and doesn't contain any artificial additives. Many lower quality CBD products are processed using toxic solvents that end up contaminating the final product. Look for a high-quality company that has every batch tested by a third party. The proof is in the test results. Any company can make purity claims but you want to make sure that they have hard science to prove it.

3) WHAT ARE THE THC LEVELS?

It's extremely important that you look for a product that has very low levels of THC, the psychoactive component that makes you high. Federal regulations demand that full-spectrum hemp oil CBD products contain less than 0.3 percent THC, but even a product with only 0.3 percent THC, if taken long enough, could cause you to test positive for marijuana. Other companies that don't test their product might have one batch under 0.3 percent and another that is much higher. They aren't doing it intentionally but not all companies have good quality control. Ideally, try to look for a product that has zero percent THC. No one wants to risk getting fired because they flunked a random drug test, especially if you are an airline pilot, police officer, nurse, truck driver, or have a job where you are subjected to regular drug tests. You do not want to put your job at risk.

4) WHAT IS THE ABSORBABILITY?

As mentioned earlier, since the human body is primarily water, CBD oil is not well absorbed. Most products on the market are absorbed at 3-6 percent. That means that most of the product is wasted—it passes directly through your system without your body absorbing most of it. That is why you want to find a water-soluble product with a high absorption rate—ideally 80-94 percent. Again, any company can claim to have high absorption rates but they should be able to prove their claims with science. The product I use at my clinic performed a very high-quality human study at an extremely reputable lab. In this absorbability study they measured the serum or blood levels of CBD absorbed by the test subjects for 12 hours to confirm their absorption claims of 80-94 percent.

5) IS IT COST EFFECTIVE?

Cost effectiveness goes hand in hand with absorption because if your body absorbs a higher percentage of the product, you are getting good value for your money. Let's break it down from a financial standpoint: If you spend $100 on a product that is absorbed at six percent, only six dollars of actual CBD oil is being absorbed by your body. When you buy a high-quality product absorbed at 80-94 percent, the maximum value is $80 to $94 per $100. When patients show me a product and try to explain how it has more oil per bottle and is cheaper than what I provide, I explain how they are comparing apples and oranges. The bottle might be bigger and cheaper, but you're only absorbing 6 percent of the CBD at best so the product is actually more expensive.

6) IS THE PRODUCT A FULL-SPECTRUM HEMP OIL?

Some CBD oils on the market are CBD isolates, which means they isolate just one fraction of the full oil. Remember that CBD isn't just one compound—there are 45 to 60 different CBD compounds. When you isolate something in the natural world and take it away from the whole, you increase potential side effects while decreasing effectiveness. This is especially the case with CBD oil.

Full-spectrum hemp oil CBD contains not only phytocan-nabinoids but it also contains terpenes. If you're familiar with essential oils, terpenes are what give essential oils their smell, healing properties, and absorbability. The terpenes have some cannabinoid effects and also potentiate or in-crease the effectiveness of the CBD compounds.

Flavonoids are another component of a full-spectrum product. Flavonoids are natural antioxidants found in other plants, even red wine and green tea, which help to drive down levels of oxidative stress. Add to that the vitamins, minerals, omegas, and essential fats, and all in all, there are more than 400 active compounds in full-spectrum hemp oil CBD that work together. The whole is far greater than the sum of the part, and nature intended for this plant to be used as a whole.

IMPROVE YOUR HEALTH & YOUR WEALTH

The hemp industry is exploding along with the popularity of CBD products. Hemp is getting attention everywhere, and that presents an excellent business opportunity. I used to run the other way from multilevel marketing and direct sales companies, but in the hemp and CBD industries, a direct sales company (the one I use in my clinic) is dominating the market.

Many companies spend a lot of money on advertising with television commercials and major media to sell their products. Their products are typically manufactured, stored in a warehouse, sold to a distributor, and finally brought to the marketplace. A direct sales company means there is a company that manufactures the product and a team of individuals promotes that product. Companies like Avon, Mary Kay, and Amway have been extremely successful with this model.

Other companies have followed the social enterprise business model similar to TOMS, which donates a pair of shoes to a child in need for every pair purchased. In fact, there is a full-spectrum hemp company that takes the same approach and pays it forward by donating prenatal and multiple vitamins to individuals in need around the world.

The health and wellness use of hemp and CBD is predicted to grow by more than 700 percent in the next year, and hemp could become a multitrillion-dollar industry in the next decade. I predict that within five years the vast majority of Americans will have tried a CBD product, and many will consume it every day.

CHAPTER SEVEN

HELP FOR THOSE WITH CHRONIC PAIN

I deal with patients in pain every day as a chiropractor. I adjust their spines to help their nervous system and suggest therapeutic exercises, relaxation techniques, meditation, and nutritional supplements. Yet in my 25-year career, I've never seen any nutritional supplement have such a profound effect on my patients as CBD.

I realize that what I've seen isn't the same as a controlled, double-blind placebo study, but many of my patients have benefited since I've begun carrying the product at my clinic. It doesn't work for all of them but nothing works 100 percent of the time for all people. My personal clinical observation is that 80-90 percent of my patients who have tried CBD for different types of pain have noticed at least some benefit—and sometimes a very profound one—from adding this safe supplement to their daily routine.

THE COMPLEX NATURE OF PAIN

We all experience pain differently but we don't always think about what is happening in the body. What we often describe as pain is actually a brain response. Our perception of pain is how we interpret a stimulus. Touching a hot stove is a thermal stimulus while stepping on a tack is a mechanical stimulus. What we call nociception is when this stimulus is sent through nerves to the spinal cord and then to the brain.

This is important to point out because this response is not the exact equivalent of what we call "pain." Someone could put their hand on a hot stove and reflexively pull away before pain even registers in their brain. This feedback loop of nociception is controlled by the nervous system. We don't register pain until the message reaches a part of the brain called the thalamus, which sends the signals to the rest of the brain, including the frontal cortex (the thinking part of the brain) and the limbic system (the emotional part of the brain and its response to pain).

Dozens of people can experience the same transmission of information but their responses can be very different. In other words, the same level of stimulus will not cause the same level of pain in all people because their brains perceive it in different ways. Pain isn't as simple as most people think. Neither is the treatment of pain.

It's important to note the goal is never to get rid of pain because it's an essential process in the body that protects us from injury. It's a warning system. An alarm. If you touch a hot stove, you know to pull your hand away. If you didn't do that, you'd do more damage to your hand. When you have back pain from nerve irritation, or even a stomach ulcer, that pain is a warning signal. It's your body telling you that there is a problem. You don't want to ignore that alarm because it often gets worse. The problem with pain, particularly chronic pain, is that your brain adapts and becomes more sensitive to pain. People with chronic pain often have a stronger response to pain than people who don't.

HOW DOES CBD HELP WITH PAIN?

One of the main reasons why patients turn to cannabinoids is to help reduce pain. The reason that it works so well is that CBD affects how pain is transmitted. A study in the *British Journal of Pharmacology* in August 1999[11] says CBD has a dampening effect on the transmission of pain through the spinal cord and to the brain.

This study on nerve pain was done on rats, not humans. (Rats and mice are often used during the initial stages of research until it is proven to be safe on animals.) Another 2007 study[12] looked at how CBD impacted chronic pain and inflammation in the sciatic nerve of rats. The rats were

---

11 Chapman V., "The Cannabinoid CB1 receptor antagonist, SR141716A, selectively facilitates nociceptive responses of dorsal horn neurons in the rat," *British Journal of Pharmacology,* 1999, Aug; 127 (8): 1765-7.
12 Costa B, Trovato AE, Comelli F, Giagnoni G, Colleoni M, "The non-psychoactive cannabis constituent cannabidiol is an orally effective therapeutic agent in rat chronic inflammatory and neuropathic pain," *European Journal of Pharmacology,* 2007 Feb 5;556(1-3); 75-83. EPUB 2006 Nov 10.

given daily oral treatment with CBD, and researchers found there was a reduction in the chemicals that indicate pain. Both of these studies are significant because they suggest that CBD can affect the transmission of pain through the spinal cord and also reduce the chemical response that transmits pain to the brain.

Cannabinoids also can impact how the brain perceives pain. During a study published in *Pain* in January 2013[13], researchers administered cannabinoids to 15 patients and then had the patients undergo functional MRIs. These are different from typical MRIs and allow researchers to see which part of the brain is working. In this case, they could see a change in the right amygdala, the deep part of the brain that is associated with pain, especially the fear aspect of pain. The amygdala is activated when we are fearful about something, and cannabinoids are effective in reducing the unpleasantness (not necessarily the intensity) of pain. Not only can cannabinoids impact the transmission of pain signals they also can change how the brain perceives pain, meaning it reduces pain by two separate mechanisms.

Other studies show how cannabinoids can help with joint pain[14] and knee pain associated with osteoarthritis[15].

13 Lee, Michael C., Ploner, Markus., Wiech, Katja., Ulrike, Bingel., Wanigasekera, Vishvarani., Brooks, Jonathan., Menon, David K., Tracey, Irene., "Amygdala activity contributes to the dissociative effect of cannabis on pain perception," *Pain.*, 2013 Jan; 154 (1): 124-134.

14 Miller RJ, Miller RE, "Is cannabis an effective treatment for joint pain," *Clinical and Experimental Rheumatology,* 2017 Sept-Oct; 35 Suppl 107 (5) 59-67. EPUB 2017 Sep 28.

15 Burston JJ, Sagar DR, Shao P, Bai M, King E, Brailsford L, Turner JM, Hathaway GJ, Bennett AJ, Walsh DA, Kendall DA, Lichtman A, Chapman V, "Cannabinoid CB2 receptors regulate central sensitization and pain responses associated with osteoarthritis of the knee joint," *PLOS One,* Nov 25;8 (11): e80440. Doi: 10.137/journal.pone.0080440. eCollection 2013.

Osteoarthritis of the knee joint is a common condition accompanied by chronic and debilitating pain. Often when people suffer from chronic pain, their brain and the nervous system becomes hypersensitive to the pain, meaning they actually feel the pain more the longer they suffer from it. The study found evidence that activation of one of the cannabinoid receptors (CB2 to be specific) in animals reduces or prevents the pain at the level of the brain (central sensitization). In doing so, it reduces chronic osteoarthritic pain.

I'm careful when using the words "all," "always," "none," and "never," but since research shows how CBD can help improve the transmission and recognition of pain within the brain and body, it's likely CBD can be effective in treating many different types of pain.

ALL DRUGS HAVE SIDE EFFECTS

Most people with minor pain pop an Advil or Tylenol without even thinking. You can buy it at the store so it has to be safe, right? Advil is ibuprofen, which is a nonsteroidal anti-inflammatory drug. It works by blocking the production of prostaglandins, a substance released in the body in response to injury that can lead to pain, swelling, and inflammation. What a lot of people don't realize is that something as seemingly harmless as Advil can lead to heartburn and, more serious, stomach bleeding. Thousands of Americans die each year from stomach bleeding due to overuse of nonsteroidal anti-inflammatory drugs[16]. Even fewer people realize there is a potential risk of asthma, liver problems, kidney problems, heart failure, and even stroke.

Tylenol is acetaminophen, a pain reliever and fever reducer believed to reduce the number of prostaglandins in the brain associated with inflammation and swelling. Tylenol may be safer for those with stomach issues. But it still can cause serious side effects like skin reactions, kidney damage, anemia, and liver damage.

The advantage of CBD is that it doesn't work by just blocking the prostaglandin pathway. It lessens the chemical response and transmission of pain without any of the possible side effects of common over-the-counter medications. A 2008 study published in *Therapeutics and Clinical Risk Management*[17] specifically looked at how cannabinoids can help with pain resulting from rheumatoid arthritis, multiple sclerosis, and cancer.

"Numerous randomized clinical trials have demonstrated safety and efficacy for the use of cannabinoids for the treatment of these pain conditions," the study abstract concludes. "The cannabinoid analgesics have usually been well tolerated in clinical trials with acceptable adverse event profiles."

What they mean when they say "well tolerated with accept-

---

16 *Nutrition Digest*, Published by the American Nutrition Association, "Deadly NSAIDs," Volume 38, No. 2.
17 Russo, Ethan B., "Cannabinoids in the management of difficult to treat pain," *Therapeutics and Clinical Risk Management*, 2008 Feb; 4(1): 245-259.

able adverse event profiles" is that the patients kept using CBD because they didn't suffer any significant side effects. In other words, the downside was minimal.

OPIOIDS AND ADDICTION

Individuals suffering from chronic pain or more severe conditions may be prescribed opioids like Vicodin, hydrocodone, codeine, or OxyContin. These are pain-relieving drugs that muffle the perception of pain. The big problem with these drugs is that they are incredibly addictive and symptoms of addiction can appear in less than three days. And withdrawal from opioids requires detox in most cases.

In March 2018, the National Institute of Drug Abuse reported that more than 115 people die in the United States every day after overdosing on opioids. The Center for Disease Control estimates that the economic burden of prescription opioid misuse in the United States is $78.5 billion a year, which includes the costs associated with healthcare, addiction treatment, low productivity, and the involvement of the criminal justice system.

What's particularly interesting is that the mechanism by which opioids reduce pain seems to be similar to CBD. If you have a choice between using an addictive opioid that can potentially have disastrous side effects, why choose that drug when there is a safe, natural compound with multiple modes of action but without the side effects or addictive qualities?

Unlike THC, CBD doesn't have psychoactive qualities or abuse potential. CBD is also proven to be a viable treatment option for a variety of symptoms associated with drug addiction. A study published in *Neurotherapeutics* in October 2015[18] looked at the preclinical animal and human studies associated with the medical use of CBD and addiction. While THC seems to increase your reward (drug-seeking) behavior, anxiety, and sensitivity to other addictive drugs, CBD seems to have the opposite effect.

This study also cited previous rat studies that showed CBD reduced heroin use and addictive behavior in rats. CBD showed a decrease in heroin cravings 24 hours after the first dose of CBD and up to seven days after the final CBD dose. These results were compared to rats given a placebo that did not have the same effect.

BACK PAIN DISAPPEARS

Consider the experience of Dr. Derrick Hendricks:

"The MRI showed I had two bulging discs in my back pushing on the nerves. The pain was excruciating and, as it got worse, it impacted my work and made adjusting patients difficult. It wasn't long before I caught myself holding my breath every time I had to push down or twist a patient.

18 Hurd YL, Yoon M, Manini AF, Hernandez S, Olmedo R, Ostman M, Jutras-Aswad D, "Early Phase in the Development of Cannabidiol as a Treatment for Addiction: Opioid Relapse Takes Initial Center Stage," *Neurotherapeutics*, 2015 Oct; 12 (4): 807-15 doi: 10.1007/s13311-015-0373-7.

I got used to living with the pain, and I subconsciously anticipated that pain. At first, I didn't even realize it.

"I started to avoid doing many things I loved out of fear of reinjuring my back. I own a small farm and always worked outside, but simple tasks like picking up hay or carrying wood became difficult—never mind the labor-intensive tasks I'd done for years. I had to get help from my kids.

"I couldn't sit still, either. I had to move constantly. If I sat down for too long, the pain got worse. The only relief I found came when I either curled up in a fetal position or placed myself over a stability ball on my stomach with my back flexed.

"I tried everything. I did decompression therapy, took medication, and went to physical therapy but the pain kept getting worse. I also turned for regular adjustments to a friend and colleague whom I've known since chiropractic school but that didn't help, either.

"At a conference at the University of Notre Dame, I heard a presentation by one of my colleagues, a fellow chiropractor from the Indianapolis area. He spoke about a miraculous new supplement he started using called CBD. I was skeptical and thought it was just snake oil. But with the pain I had, I also felt desperate so I gave it a try.

"The first thing I noticed after taking CBD was that I slept like a baby. It happened within a day or two of taking my first dose. I hadn't slept like that in years—probably not since I was a teenager. My back pain didn't go away but I slept through the night and woke up feeling refreshed. If I hadn't gotten that result, I might have stopped. It wasn't until I had taken the supplement every single day for about two months that I realized the pain in my back was gone. Not a little bit better or 50 percent better—completely gone.

"I noticed it for the first time when I was in my office and no longer had to hold my breath and brace myself before adjusting a patient. I could work on the farm again. I could split wood and do all the heavy lifting I had delegated to my kids.

"Before taking CBD, I convinced myself my condition was not only going to be permanent but that it was going to get progressively worse and severely limit my mobility as I got older. Not a day went by when I didn't worry about that. This product was literally life-changing.

"Now, I recommend CBD to all my patients for a multitude of problems. I continue to be amazed on almost a daily basis by the results they get from CBD."

A HUSBAND AND WIFE GET THEIR HEALTH BACK

This is what Valerie Mullikin says about CBD:

"My husband, Steve, is a veteran of the United States Navy and served in Operation Desert Storm in 1991. He is now 100 percent disabled due to a demyelinating disease that is currently listed as atypical primary progressive multiple sclerosis with autonomic dysfunction.

"When he began to experience numbness and mild paralysis in 1991, the Navy didn't know what was wrong, so they ran some tests and discovered he had a demyelinating disease of the white matter all over his brain. The doctor's exact words were: 'Your brain lights up like a Christmas tree.'

"The doctor sent my husband for an MRI and a spinal tap, but both came back perfectly normal. All of his blood work came back completely normal so they sent us to the National Institutes of Health. We were then sent to Massachusetts General. We were sent to Johns Hopkins. We were sent to the Cleveland Clinic. We were sent to the Mayo Clinic. We were sent to Ohio State University, the University of Cincinnati, the University of Indiana, and my husband's spinal fluid, blood work, and MRIs were sent to three other international medical facilities. Nobody could tell us what was wrong with him.

"About 15 years ago, my husband suffered his first bout of trigeminal neuralgia on the right side of his face. That resulted in five PSR brain surgeries to address the trigeminal nerve that was attacking all three branches on the right side of his face. That resulted in additional numbness to his face but it was manageable. My husband was on quite a few prescription drugs.

"Meanwhile, I experienced chronic pain in my chest. My sternum hurt when I pressed on it. I went to see my primary care doctor who conducted lab work and tests. I had everything done except for a cardiac catheterization and nothing showed up. I did my own research and my doctor thought that I might have costochondritis, which involves inflammation of muscles in the chest cavity.

"My doctor suggested CBD. She said that if I experienced any relief within 48 hours to give her a call and she would give me a bottle. About 24 hours later, I gave her a call and asked how I could get it. I had not researched the product or the company—I was just willing to give it a try. A month later, my bottle finally came in, and I experienced great relief as soon as I started taking it.

"The CBD worked so well for me that I recommended it to my husband. He took one dose and that night when we were sleeping, his body stopped moving. At first, I thought he was dead because his body never stops moving when he sleeps. He runs, flails, hits, and rolls, but that night he didn't move, and that was one of the best nights of sleep I have had in 20 years. My husband took my little sample bottle and used it. He realized he felt refreshed when he woke up in the morning.

"The following month, he suffered another bout of trigeminal neuralgia to the left side of his face. We were not prepared for this. It was absolutely devastating for us. As soon as it happened, I convinced him to take a second dose of CBD. He set his timer and it took 19 minutes for the trigeminal neuralgia to resolve.

"My husband now faithfully takes his CBD twice a day, every 12 hours, and he never misses a dose. Since August 2018, he has been pain free and without any of the heavy prescription drugs he was taking—oral steroids, Gabapentin, Dilantin, Baclofen, and Aspirin. He stayed on his blood pressure medication to address the autonomic dysfunction in his body, which, by the way, is at its lowest dose ever. We're eager to see what the new MRI shows and how he continues to improve because he's experiencing great improvements already.

"We've also noticed his moods have balanced, his sleep has improved, the trigeminal neuralgia is under control, and he's not fatigued like he used to be. It's exciting and we're hoping that our testimony can help another veteran.

"Meanwhile, the CBD has helped to reduce the pain in my chest cavity dramatically. I no longer feel that pain like I once did, thank God. It's tolerable and no longer crippling. I know this is working. It will just take some time. CBD is nothing short of a miracle for us, and we know that it can be the same for others."

THE LIFE-CHANGING EFFECT OF CBD

This is the story of Melissa Sones:

"I've battled chronic pain since I was in two car accidents, the first in 2003 and the second in 2004. Debilitating pain robbed me of who I am, my career, and time with my family.

"I'm thankful I have a very loving and supportive spouse who has been by my side through it all. He kept things going when I could not. We met with doctors and I was put on countless medications, some helped but were never enough. Some medications came with side effects like weight gain, depression, and loss of cognitive ability.

"In late September 2018, it was by chance I commented on a Facebook post—something I rarely do. I talked with a friend and she offered me a trial of CBD. After doing some research, I agreed. I began using CBD and within three days noticed amazing results. I experienced a dramatic decrease in pain and was able to do things I haven't done in years. I felt so much better. I slept more soundly.

"As I continued using CBD, I noticed more and more benefits. I have mental clarity and the ability to focus. My anxiety decreased, my blood sugar is easier to regulate, I've lost weight, and, most important, my mood has significantly improved.

"CBD has been life-changing. I have wanted to shout from the rooftops to everyone I know about it. It's not just about chronic pain. The benefits go so far beyond pain, and I experienced all of this after only taking the product for one month.

"This is the single most promising thing that we have found to help since we began this journey with chronic pain and other health struggles. This is such an exciting time in our lives. And contrary to the misconception, CBD is not a drug—it's a THC-free oil that is legal in all 50 states."

CHAPTER EIGHT

ALLEVIATE ANXIETY AND DEPRESSION IN DAYS

Many people struggle on a daily basis with physical pain or emotional pain, to varying degrees. With my patients, I spend a lot of time sharing ideas and solutions to help them experience less physical and emotional pain and enjoy more peace in their lives. CBD is a great tool to help my patients in all of these areas.

AN UNEXPECTED RESULT

One of the blessings of being a chiropractor is that I get to develop very personal relationships with my patients. I consider many of my patients as family. Some of them don't suffer from any pain at all and just come in so I can adjust their spine to optimize the function of their nervous system which promotes health as opposed to treating disease. This preventative approach is the best way to benefit from chiropractic care and has traditionally been the paradigm of chiropractors. The old saying that "an ounce of prevention is worth a pound of cure" is very true when it comes to our health.

John was a different type of patient. He suffered from a lower back disc herniation that caused him severe lower back and leg pain. He responded well to my treatment but the response was slow given the severity of his condition. Eventually, we got rid of about 90 percent of his pain but some of it lingered. John was active. He kayaked, hiked, and did a lot of other outdoor activities in addition to having a physically demanding job. He was anxious to improve his condition.

I experienced such great results with CBD myself that I told John there was a good chance it might help with his back pain. With most of my patients, I suggest they try it for one month to see how it works for them and I recommended that John do the same thing. When he arrived for his appointment the following week, I asked him about the CBD.

He looked me right in the eye and said with a serious voice, "Doc, I will never stop taking this product."

That surprised me. "What happened? Does your back feel that much better?"

"No. I mean, it's helped a little with my back, but by the second day, I noticed a huge improvement in this severe anxiety that I didn't even tell you I had," he said. "That has completely disappeared."

John went on to explain how he suffered from anxiety for years. It affected his job, his social life, his ability to relax, and especially his sleep. All those problems started to improve almost immediately after taking the CBD. What surprised me the most about John's story was how he unintentionally discovered such a valuable benefit. I had known John for years so I was overjoyed for him. It's wonderful when I can help my patients in such a safe and natural way.

Since John's experience with CBD, I've witnessed other patients experience similar results. I've had patients tell me that CBD has been "life-changing," and I have witnessed firsthand how CBD has helped patients deal with their anxiety—something I didn't initially realize was a benefit of taking CBD.

WHAT DOES THE SCIENCE PROVE?

While doing my research, I found an interesting study in *Neurotherapeutics* that pointed to CBD's potential to treat a wide variety of anxiety and stress disorders, which is a profound discovery.

"We found that existing preclinical evidence strongly supports CBD as a treatment for generalized anxiety disorder, panic disorder, social anxiety disorder, obsessive-compulsive disorder, and posttraumatic stress disorder when administered acutely," researchers concluded in the study "Cannabidiol as a Potential Treatment for Anxiety

Disorders."[19] "However, few studies have investigated chronic CBD dosing."

If CBD only helped with these conditions alone it would truly be considered miraculous but it's even more miraculous to consider its additional benefits.

As I previously mentioned, the reason why CBD has these effects is that it contains phytocannabinoids that naturally enhance the human body's endocannabinoid system. But why does it help so much with anxiety and depression? It's worth noting that nerves in the brain and spinal cord are rich with these receptors, specifically those commonly referred to as CB1 receptors that allow CBD to positively affect the brain.

WHAT DO PEOPLE FEAR THE MOST?

Many people cite public speaking as their number one fear, some even admit that they fear it more than death. Even those who don't have social anxiety disorder often say that they fear having to speak in public more than anything else. So, what better way to test the effects of CBD on anxiety than placing people in one of the most stressful situations

19 Blessing, Esther M., Steenkamp, Maria M., Manzanares, Jorge., Marmar, Charles R., "Cannabidiol as a Potential Treatment for Anxiety Disorders," *Neurotherapeutics*, 2015 Oct; 12(4): 825-836.

possible? This is precisely what researchers did in a 2011 study.[20]

What's so interesting about this study is that it involved patients who suffered from social anxiety disorder and also people who didn't suffer from any anxiety. It specifically looked at one particular anxiety condition called Generalized Social Anxiety Disorder, which impairs social lives by making it difficult for people to interact with others. The point of the study was to look at how CBD influenced both sets of patients.

This was a double-blind study, which is considered to be a higher quality study because researchers don't just look at one side—in this case, the beneficial effect of CBD. The patients were split into two groups (hence double) with a mix in both groups of patients who suffered from anxiety and those who didn't. The first group was given a dose of CBD and the second group was given a placebo. What makes the study "blind" is that neither group knows which compound they are getting. This is crucial because the placebo effect (the effect of people taking something and getting better, even if it's just a sugar pill) makes a difference.

Our brain controls how our body works, so when people just think that they are taking something that will help them, they can get better even if they aren't taking anything

20 Mateus M Bergamaschi, Regina Helena Costa Queiroz, Marcos Hortes Nisihara Chagas, Danielle Chaves Gomes de Oliveira, Bruno Spinosa De Martinis, Flávio Kapczinski, João Quevedo, Rafael Roesler, Nadja Schröder, Antonio E Nardi, Rocio Martín-Santos, Jaime Eduardo Cecílio Hallak, Antonio Waldo Zuardi, and José Alexandre S. Crippa, "Cannabidiol Reduces the Anxiety Induced by Simulated Public Speaking in Treatment-Naïve Social Phobia Patients," *Neuropsychopharmacology,* 2011 May; 36(6) 1219-1226.

beneficial. In this study, researchers were able to study people under the same conditions to help determine how much of the benefit was due to the CBD.

Once the compounds were administered, each patient was subjectively rated during a simulated public speaking test using a visual analog mood scale, which is a standard assessment using pictures showing faces with expressions ranging from sad to happy. They also were rated according to a negative self-statement scale, which is a series of questions to rate the experience in terms of its negativity. Researchers also monitored blood pressure, heart rate, and skin conductance. This was all measured at six different times throughout the public speaking test. The participants also completed a questionnaire after the study.

When researchers analyzed the results, they found those treated with CBD experienced significantly reduced anxiety, cognitive impairment (inability to focus and speak), and overall discomfort. Significantly decreased alert levels (nervousness about public speaking) were experienced both by those with anxiety and those without.

Meanwhile, the placebo group, which did not receive anything, exhibited higher anxiety, discomfort, and higher alert levels under the same set of circumstances compared with those who were given CBD.

A SAFE ALTERNATIVE

Every drug has side effects but that is especially true for antidepressants and antianxiety drugs, some of which are known to cause suicidal/homicidal thoughts and actions. As a result, the FDA has placed a "Black Box" label on these drugs—the most serious type of warning on prescription drug labeling. Many natural health experts believe that these prescriptions often do more harm than good.

Even though medications are sometimes necessary, my goal as a chiropractor is to work with my patients and their medical doctors to reduce their dependence on pharmaceutical drugs and present them with healthy and safe alternatives. We've talked about side effects but the dangers of prescriptions drugs go well beyond the side effects.

The sad reality is that we as a society have grown completely numb even to "Black Box" warnings. Think of all the television commercials for pharmaceutical drugs. Often, it takes longer to list the side effects than it does the remedies. My own children, who probably have a different perspective having grown up in a natural chiropractic family ask, "Dad, why would anybody want to take that medication?" The sad truth is that some people are living in so much pain that they are willing to risk serious side effects and even death to treat an ailment.

The unfortunate reality is that some people experience such severe anxiety and depression that they take their own lives. It is estimated that an average of 22 veterans, many of whom experience posttraumatic stress disorder (PTSD), commit suicide every day. In the 2015 study cited previously, PTSD is one of the conditions listed as being treatable with CBD, and CBD has been shown to help.

JUST BECAUSE IT'S A DRUG DOESN'T MEAN IT'S BETTER

There is one story that I have been telling my patients for years that is based on a couple of different studies.[21, 22] I share it with them to bring home the point that natural treatments can sometimes be more effective and safer than prescription drugs.

I start with telling them about researchers who studied three different groups of women with clinical depression. The first group took an antidepressant. The second group took an antidepressant and were instructed to take three 20-minute walks per week. The third group was instructed only to walk for 20 minutes three times a week. After following each group of women over a period of time, researchers determined that the group that only did the walking exhibited the most significant reduction in anxiety and stress while also experiencing the fewest relapses. Something as simple as walking an hour a week proved to be more beneficial

---

21 Craft, Lynette L., Perna, Frank M., "The Benefits of Exercise for the Clinically Depressed," *The Primary Care Companion to the Journal of Clinical Psychiatry*, 2004; 6(3): 104-111.
22 Heesch KC, van Gellecum YR, Burton NW, van Uffelen JG, Brown WJ, "Physical activity, walking, and quality of life in women with depressive symptoms," *American Journal of Preventative Medicine*, 2015 Mar;48(3): 281-91. EPUB 2015 Jan 13.

than prescription medication, even if it was combined with walking.

I'm not disparaging prescription drugs nor am I recommending that people stop using correctly prescribed medications. Some drugs can save people's lives and are absolutely necessary, but my point is that a safe treatment alternative with fewer side effects should be considered. As the negative side effects of medication become more well known, the wiser it seems to look for a drug-free approach.

Most of my patients experience the full health benefits of CBD after taking the product correctly for two months. But one of the most amazing things I've noticed is that 80-90 percent of my patients experience a rapid response. They report a decrease in their levels of anxiety and depression after using the product only for a day or two—and some of the results are dramatic. I've even had patients experience a sense of relief and peace only minutes after taking their first dose.

Taking a dose of CBD throughout the day during intense moments of stress and anxiety has been able to quell potential anxiety attacks in some patients. As important, these patients all experience relief without any side effects or risk of dependency.

A VETERAN IS SAVED FROM SUICIDE

This is what Lisa Mills says about her experience with CBD:

"I joined the Air Force in 1999 and served as an aircraft mechanic before being deployed to the Middle East in 2008. I had been there for three days when an enemy rocket landed 50 feet from me and sent me flying into a concrete barrier. I suffered a traumatic brain injury and damaged my spine, which left me with PTSD upon my return to the states.

"I was put on many medications. I took a nonsteroidal anti-inflammatory, a steroid anti-inflammatory, muscle relaxers to deal with spasms, antidepressants, sedatives, compound creams, pain patches to put on my skin, a relaxant, drugs for migraines, drugs for nerve pain, bipolar disorder, and even anti-smoking drugs.

"On top of all the meds, I wore back braces, went to physical therapy, used a TENS unit (transcutaneous electrical nerve stimulation), which came with electrodes you hook up to your body so your muscles tense and release, and also used an RS-4i Plus, which works out your muscles and does the same thing as a TENS but times a thousand.

The majority of the drugs I took were opioids (even though people addicted to prescription opioids have a 40-60 percent higher risk of suicide).

"My injuries took their toll on me and so did the medication. I had a loving family and supportive friends but I still felt alone and unworthy of love and affection. A few days before my oldest child turned two, I survived my third suicide attempt. I wrestled with suicidal thoughts until May

2018. That's when I was introduce to CBD and everything changed.

"Now, I take no medication. I only take CBD. That's it. I noticed a change three days after taking the product. I had more energy and focus and I haven't had a single suicidal thought. I can play with my two kids now, whereas only a few months before taking the product I couldn't sit on the floor with them. I couldn't ride a bike. The product has changed my life by giving me back my life."

DEPRESSION IS LIFTED

Consider what Maranda Siewert has to say about CBD:

"I had been suffering from depression for years but it wasn't until January 2018 when I was officially diagnosed. It came after I was hospitalized for five days at Rogers Memorial Hospital in Oconomowoc, Wisconsin. The psychiatrist put me on an SSRI type of antidepressant medication, Lexapro, to help with the symptoms of depression.

"Once I was discharged, the eating disorder I'd struggled with since I was a teenager intensified. I tried to hide it from my family, but eventually, they noticed how much weight I lost so I was placed in a partial hospitalization program where I worked with dietitians. My family got increasingly upset and frustrated with me so I isolated myself. The isolation fueled my depression. It was a cycle.

"Meanwhile, I continued to work with all kinds of therapists and a nurse practitioner who helped manage all the meds that I took for my depression. On top of that, they added an antipsychotic in an attempt to manage the suicidal thoughts. Nothing seemed to work.

"I felt hopeless. I was at rock bottom. A family member suggested I try CBD to help with my symptoms. I bought a bottle and applied one dropper of the oil under my tongue. In one hour, I began to feel like my old self. At first, my mom didn't believe me. She thought I was faking it. But I convinced her to try it and she eventually saw the results for herself as it helped with her own anxiety.

"Over time, my symptoms settled, as did the way I felt about food. All of those feelings and urges that used to cripple me were less intense. Today, I don't want to isolate myself in my room or spend my days sleeping or watching television alone. I don't have the desire to restrict my food or purge. More importantly, my mood is better.

"CBD doesn't just make me feel better; I can see the impact my mood has on my family. I know for a fact that CBD is responsible for the improvement. When I don't take it or miss a dose, my mood changes and I slip back into my old thought patterns. I still take prescription medication but I'm hoping to wean myself off all my meds and eventually only take the CBD."

CHAPTER NINE

A NATURAL WAY TO COMBAT DIABETES

I have been simply amazed at the success many people have had with CBD and Donn Rudd is no exception.

Donn is a 71 year old veteran who suffers from diabetes and arthritis. A short time ago, he was on a list at the Veterans Administration (VA) waiting for a knee replacement but his health problems started to escalate after he suffered a heart attack. Three of his arteries were 100 percent blocked and too small for stents to be inserted. Instead, doctors put Donn on nine different cardiac medications. Since he was diabetic, the medications caused his blood sugar levels to skyrocket from its normal range of 120 to 150 up to 230 and eventually all the way up to 380. That was so high and the damage to his kidneys so severe that the VA refused his knee replacement surgery.

Running out of options, Donn looked into chelation therapy (an IV treatment used to remove heavy metals from the bloodstream.) First, however, his doctor tested his heart to see if it was strong enough for the therapy. Three days later, Donn was told he had Stage 3 kidney disease, one stage before dialysis is necessary. Diabetes and the heart medication were killing his kidneys, but he didn't see dialysis as an option.

"I'm not doing it," Donn told his wife Sherry. "I saw the way your dad suffered on dialysis. You lose your life and ability to do anything."

He told me, "God is bigger than I am. I can't handle this, but God can."

I think God has a plan for all of us, too, and I believe that's what happened with Donn. Two days later, Donn was invited to attend a CBD meeting. He heard so many stories about its incredible results that Donn immediately got a bottle of CBD oil and began using it.

Earlier that day, Donn's blood sugar level tested at 230. That night, he took his first dose of CBD. In the morning, he checked his blood sugar, and much to his shock, it was 99. Donn hadn't seen that number in 20 years. His first reaction was that it was too good to be true, so he poked himself in a different finger, and once again the test came back: 99. He was so amazed and excited that he woke up his wife.

Donn went to the VA monthly to get his blood checked and receive his A1c score, which monitors his long-term blood sugar levels. Three weeks before using CBD every day, his score came back as 9.9, which was very high. The next time he went to have his blood tested, the doctor was amazed that his score had dropped from 9.9 to 7.9.

Donn pulled out the bottle of CBD oil and said, "It must be from this."

The doctor looked at it and said, "This is just a supplement. It's not FDA approved. It couldn't possibly be this."

"Well, those nine cardiac meds you put me on, those were FDA approved," Donn replied, "and they aren't doing squat for me."

Still, at the doctor's request, Donn stopped using the CBD oil for several days. The next time he checked his blood sugar at home, it had climbed back up to dangerously high levels, so he went back to using the CBD oil every day.

A month later, he returned to the VA for his regular blood test and this time the doctor was even more amazed to see that his A1c had dropped all the way down to 6.2. That's a remarkable score for someone who had been as high as 9.9 only two months earlier.

"Maybe you should just keep using that CBD oil," the doctor said.

Donn continues to maintain control of his blood sugar levels by using the CBD oil. They even dropped low enough for the VA to approve his knee replacement. What's funny is that since Donn had been using the CBD oil, not only did he lower his blood sugar but he found his knee wasn't bothering him anymore. He opted not to have the knee replacement.

I tell this story about Donn because it highlights what I see in my practice. I've recommended patients take CBD for arthritis and knee problems only to learn a short time later it caused their blood sugar levels to drop and allowed them to take fewer medications to manage their diabetes. In other words, Donn isn't an isolated case and his results are not unusual.

We don't know much about CBD and how it affects the pancreas, inflammation, and diabetes, and more research is needed. It would be huge news if a natural plant product helped control diabetes and diminished secondary kidney and skin problems associated with the disease. It could save lives, limit suffering, and reduce medical costs for a growing health problem nationwide.

HOW DOES DIABETES AFFECT YOUR BODY?

Simply put, diabetes is the body's inability to properly process sugar. This leads to high blood sugar levels that can be extremely damaging to vital organs. Diabetes can lead to nerve damage in the feet and hands and also to diabetes-related dementia, as well as kidney failure, which can be fatal.

There are two types of diabetes: Type 1 and type 2. Type 1 is primarily thought to be an autoimmune disease resulting from damage to the part of the pancreas that produces insulin. Pancreatic islets, or islets of Langerhans, are the part of the pancreas that secrete the hormone insulin and help your body maintain proper levels of sugar in the blood. Insulin is released in response to your diet by what's called the beta cells (or B-cells) in the islets of Langerhans.

No one knows for certain what leads to type 1 diabetes but there is nearly always inflammation and damage done to the B-cells. Until we discovered the benefits of CBD, there was not much you could do to treat type 1 diabetes except for medication to artificially maintain blood sugar levels.

Type 2 diabetes is primarily caused by lifestyle and diet, and it's close to becoming an epidemic. Not only are people eating more foods high in sugar and starches but they consume soda and processed foods that contain a highly concentrated form of sugar called high-fructose corn syrup. A lack of regular physical exercise also can contribute to diabetes. The good news is that Type 2 diabetes is treatable and can even be reversed with changes in diet and exercise. CBD can be a huge help, too.

Type 2 diabetes is often preceded by insulin resistance, which means that the insulin your body produces becomes less and less effective. The more you consume a diet high in sugar and the more your blood sugar goes up, the more your body responds by producing insulin. If your blood sugar levels go too high or too low in either direction, it can kill you.

Let's say you eat a bunch of candy and drink a lot of soda.

This causes your blood sugar to rise and your body produces insulin. The insulin drives down those blood sugar levels so it can be absorbed into your body, processed by the liver, and ultimately stored by your body as fat. Your body begins to respond less with each sugar spike.

I ask my patients to picture a teacher trying to get control of an unruly classroom of students. The teacher raises her voice and tells them to be quiet. The first time it works, but the next time the kids just ignore her, so she has to yell louder. When it happens again, even the yelling doesn't work, so she has to blow a whistle. Pretty soon, even the whistle doesn't work, and so on. You get the idea.

This same cycle of diminishing responses happens in your body when it becomes desensitized to higher and higher levels of insulin production. Eventually, you can't keep up that level of insulin production so your blood sugar levels rise out of control.

HOW CAN CBD HELP?

Type 1 diabetes causes damage to B-cells that release insulin, and researchers have discovered that CBD decreases the damage and inflammation done to those cells.

"Evidence is emerging that some non-psychotropic plant cannabinoids, such as cannabidiol (CBD), can be employed to retard B-cell damage in type 1 diabetes," according to a 2011 study published in the *Handbook on Experimental Pharmacology*[23].

In another study published in *Autoimmunity* in 2006[24], researchers administered CBD to mice that were bred to develop diabetes. Only 30 percent of the mice treated with CBD developed diabetes, compared to 86 percent of the mice in the control group that did not receive CBD. That is a dramatic reduction. Researchers found that the mice treated with CBD experienced significantly less cell inflammation. This is significant because type 1 diabetes is an autoimmune disease where the body attacks itself and cells can become so inflamed they eventually stop producing insulin. This study suggests that CBD limits that inflammation.

Another study in *Neuropharmacology* in 2008[25] also found levels of inflammation in the pancreas were dramatically reduced in mice treated with CBD and genetically bred to develop diabetes.

"We have previously reported that cannabidiol (CBD) lowers the incidence of diabetes in young nonobese diabetes-prone (NOD) female mice," researchers reported. "In the present study, we show that administration of CBD to 11-14-week-old female NOD mice, which are either in a

23 DiMarzo V., Piscitelli F., Mechoulam R., "Cannabinoids and endocannabinoids in metabolic disorders with focus on diabetes," *Handbook on Experimental Pharmacology*, 2011; (203): 75-104.
24 Weiss, L., Zeira M., Reich S., Har-Noy M., Mechoulam R., Slavin S., Gallily R., "Cannabidiol lowers incidence of diabetes in nonobese diabetic mice," *Autoimmunity*, 2006 Mr;39(2): 143-51.
25 Weiss L., Zeira M., Reich S., Slavin S., Raz I., Mechoulam R., Gallily R., "Cannabidiol arrests onset of autoimmune diabetes in NOD mice," *Neuropharmacology*, 2008 Jan; 54(1): 244-9 EPUB 2007 Jul 17.

latent diabetes stage or with initial symptoms of diabetes, ameliorates the manifestations of the disease. Diabetes was diagnosed in only 32 percent of the mice in the CBD-treated group, compared to 86 percent and 100 percent in the emulsifier-treated and untreated groups."

This is an amazing result! Let me explain this in simpler terms. Mice that are genetically designed to develop diabetes did not develop it after they received CBD. That included mice who already showed early symptoms of the disease. The control group that did not receive CBD did not get these results. I think the most telling statement is the final sentence of the abstract: "Our data strengthen our previous assumption that CBD, known to be safe in man, can possibly be used as a therapeutic agent for treatment of type 1 diabetes."

Type 2 diabetes, if untreated, can lead to the same type of damage to your heart, blood vessels, brain, and kidneys as type 1 diabetes, but the difference is that Type 2 diabetes is preventable and reversible with lifestyle and dietary changes. Granted, those types of changes can be challenging for some people, especially later in life. However, CBD has been shown to lower blood sugar levels, often without making these types of lifestyle changes. I would argue that taking CBD along with lifestyle changes would have an even more profound effect but the CBD has proven to be effective on its own. Donn's story is the perfect example of how CBD can alter blood sugar levels without any change in diet or lifestyle. In fact, almost every patient whom I recommended take CBD noticed a reduction in their blood sugar levels.

Jane is another patient of mine who is a Type 2 diabetic. She struggles to exercise because of her joint pain. When her blood sugar levels got very high, I recommended she started taking CBD. After only three weeks, her reading dropped 40 points down to 188 without her making any other dietary changes. I've had patients who took the product for different reasons and reported back to me that they saw a drop in their blood sugar levels without making any other changes.

OXIDATIVE STRESS

Oxidative stress, which is an imbalance in your body's ability to handle free radicals, is believed to be one of the root causes of insulin resistance and B cell death. Oxidative stress can damage protein, DNA, lipids, and fats in your body. It can eventually lead to chronic diseases like athero-sclerosis, rheumatoid arthritis, heart attack, heart disease, chronic inflammation, and stroke. It's definitely something you want to avoid.

Multiple factors can cause oxidative stress, including too much sugar in your diet, infections, toxins, not getting enough sleep, and not having enough antioxidants. When people think about antioxidants, they think mainly about foods like brightly colored fruits and vegetables. But CBD is another powerful antioxidant, according to a September

2011 study[26] that found the natural compound may be useful "in treating many human diseases and disorders now known to involve activation of the immune system and associated oxidative stress...(including) rheumatoid arthritis, Types 1 and 2 diabetes, atherosclerosis, Alzheimer disease, hypertension, metabolic syndrome, ischemia-reperfusion injury, depression, and neuropathic pain."

THE COMPLICATIONS OF DIABETES

Cardiovascular disease, kidney damage, nerve damage, skin conditions, hearing impairment, and Alzheimer's disease—these are all possible complications of diabetes, and the list goes on.

One reason why CBD is so effective in treating diabetes is that it lowers high blood sugar levels that lead to changes in the lining of your blood vessels and it reduces or prevents inflammation and hardened arteries that can lead to heart attacks. CBD helps prevent the heart health risks that we typically see in diabetics, according to a 2007 study[27].

This can be a tremendous asset for early treatment and to help further prevent the various complications associated with diabetes.

---

26 Booz GW., "Cannabidiol as an emergent therapeutic strategy for lessoning the impact of inflammation on oxidative stress," *Free Radical Biology & Medicine,* 2011 Sep 1;51(5): 1054-61 EPUB 2011 Jan 14.
27 Am J Physiol Heart Circ Physiol. 2007 Jul;293(1):H610-9. EPUB 2007 Mar 23. "Cannabidiol attenuates high glucose-induced endothelial cell inflammatory response and barrier disruption."

"Our results suggest that CBD, which has recently been approved for the treatment of inflammation, pain, and spasticity associated with multiple sclerosis in humans, may have significant therapeutic benefits against diabetic complications and atherosclerosis," researchers concluded.

Conventional medicine and dieticians promotes lifestyle changes as the primary way to help avoid and combat Type 2 diabetes, but too often physicians immediately prescribe medications like Metformin to control blood sugar levels. The American Diabetes Association recommends that lifestyle interventions such as diet and exercise should be the first choice for diabetes prevention and treatment. The addition of CBD to this recommendation instead of the use of drugs could have profound benefits for patients dealing with Type 2 diabetes.

THE FATHER OF CANNABINOID RESEARCH

I want to end this chapter with an insight from Dr. Raphael Mechoulam, a research scientist from the Hebrew University of Jerusalem. He is considered the "father of cannabinoid research" because he discovered and isolated the first two cannabinoid chemicals, THC and CBD. He continues to do research, and his team still is considered one of the best in the world[28].

Dr. Mechoulam has made it clear that naturally occurring

28 *The Scientist: Are We Missing Something*, a documentary by The Canna Fundacion.
The Scientist is a documentary that traces the story of Professor Mechoulam and his pioneering work with Cannabis and the discovery of the Endocannabinoid System.

CBD receptors can be found throughout the human body—the brain, nervous system, immune system, organs, and crucially for those who suffer from diabetes, the islet cells in the pancreas. He found CBD receptors to be common in the pancreas, which produces insulin. This is critical as we know that CBD has a homeostasis or balancing effect through these receptors and controlling diabetes is all about balancing the production of insulin. Dr. Mechoulam made this discovery decades ago, but the medical and pharmaceutical industries have yet to perform large-scale human studies that could lead to the widespread use of CBD for diabetes with profound and positive consequences.

CHAPTER TEN

AT THE CORE– REDUCING INFLAMMATION

Inflammation is often considered the root cause of most disease and illness in the Western world. This becomes clear if you look at research from Harvard and Yale, among other numerous studies, that link chronic inflammation to diseases like asthma, arthritis, Crohn's disease, inflammatory bowel disease, autoimmune disease, Alzheimer's, cancer, cardiovascular disease, heart disease, diabetes, high blood pressure, high cholesterol, Parkinson's disease, joint pain, and rheumatoid arthritis. That's not even all of them.

Inflammation, however, is not always bad. It's the body's natural defense against damaged cells, viruses, and bacteria, and it's how the body triggers healing in case of damage or illness. When there is damage to the tissue, an invading microorganism or an abnormal cell in the body, the body fights it with inflammation.

Think of what happens when a cut gets infected. The area

gets red, swells, and sometimes even gets hot. That is the classic sign of inflammation, and it's how the immune system goes about attacking an infection to get rid of bacteria and restore proper function. A problem develops when that inflammation is overactive and chronic. Too much inflammation is dangerous and, unfortunately, it's all too common.

The standard medical approach to treating inflammation is with medications like nonsteroidal anti-inflammatory drugs. Steroid medications also are used to treat inflammation. But these medications come with a whole host of side effects, including hemorrhaging in the digestive system that in some cases can be fatal. A study conducted by the American Gastroenterological Association in 2005[29] claimed that approximately 16,500 people die each year from NSAIDs. During therapy with NSAIDs, patients are also at risk for renal toxicity, increased blood pressure, and increased risk of heart failure. Steroids are an even stronger anti-inflammatory that can throw off your bodily functions and should rarely be taken long term.

Given these statistics, it's no surprise that many people seek out a natural, safe, plant-based alternative to NSAIDs to control inflammation and improve their health.

Part of the reason why people find CBD helpful for different ailments is because inflammation is the root cause of so many conditions. I've witnessed it firsthand in my own

29 American Gastroenterological Association, "Study Shows Long-term Use of NSAIDs Causes Severe Intestinal Damage," *Science News,* January 14, 2005.

practice. Many of my patients who suffer from chronic inflammation in the form of joint pain, tendonitis, arthritis, autoimmune issues, chronic colitis, Crohn's disease, and inflammatory bowel problems all have responded remarkably well to this natural, safe, plant-based supplement.

What's even more remarkable is that CBD has helped patients who weren't able to get any results or find relief from over-the-counter or prescribed anti-inflammatory drugs[30].

AN ALTERNATIVE TO PHARMACEUTICALS?

Cannabinoid receptors offer an opportunity to treat inflammatory and autoimmune disorders, according to an August 2010 study[31]. I'll spare you the biochemistry, but basically, this study concluded that cannabinoids like CBD provide an alternative way of treating types of inflammatory and autoimmune disorders where the body attacks itself.

Cannabinoids suppress the inflammatory response and subsequently tend to improve disease symptoms. The study concluded by claiming that "overall, cannabinoids have a significant potential as an anti-inflammatory agent."

A similar study[32] published in 2011 also said, "CBD

30 Zoltan Varga, Syed Rafay Ali Sabzwari, and Veronika Vargova, "Cardiovascular Risk of Nonsteroidal Anti-Inflammatory Drugs: An Under-Recognized, Public Health Issue," *Cureus*, April 2017.

31 Future Medicinal Chemistry, "Cannabinoids as novel anti-inflammatory drugs" Prakash Nagarkatti,† Rupal Pandey,* Sadiye Amcaoglu Rieder,* Venkatesh L Hegde, and Mitzi Nagarkatti, https://www.ncbi.nlm.nih.gov/pmc/articles/PMC2828614/.

32 Booz, George W., "Cannabidiol as an Emergent Therapeutic Strategy for Lessening the Impact of Inflammation on Oxidative Stress," *Free Radical Biology & Medicine Journal*, 2011 Sep 1: 51(5) 1054-1061.

offers promise as a prototype for anti-inflammatory drug development."

What baffles me is that instead of using a safe and effective natural product, pharmaceutical companies try to create a drug that duplicates that natural product. Why not just take the natural product? The sad truth is that it's all about money.

You can't patent a natural product, and there is not a lot of money to be made selling natural products compared to the money that can be made on a patented drug[33]. However, attempts to replicate or make a synthetic version of a natural product will almost always be more likely to cause side effects. Your body knows what to do with natural foods and plants, but synthetic or artificial versions of a natural plant are chemically different. The human body already makes endogenous or natural cannabinoids, plus our bodies can use a nutrient-like, full-spectrum hemp or CBD to prevent a deficiency in the endocannabinoid system, which influences so many functions in the human body.

The science doesn't lie, and both of these studies suggest CBD is useful in the treatment of numerous diseases and disorders from diabetes and Alzheimer's disease to hypertension and neuropathic pain. These may seem like very different diseases and conditions but the common denominator is that almost all of them are tied to inflammation.

33 Harvard Journal of Law & Technology, Volume 30, Number 2 Spring 2017, "Patenting Natural Products After Myriad," Evan H. Tallmadge.

INTESTINAL INFLAMMATION

When I was in school 25 years ago, we were taught that you were born with a certain amount of brain cells that died off as you aged. As a result, it was assumed your brain function would decline with age. We now know that it is completely untrue.

Your body still produces new cells whether you're two, 10, 50, or 100 years old. It's whether those brain cells are stimulated that determines whether they add to your brain function or merely fade away. In particular, the glial cells in the brain maintain its balance and support the nervous system. The word "glial" actually comes from the word "glue."

These glial cells also are found in the intestines, and cutting-edge research increasingly describes the gut as a kind of second brain[34]. All of your combined systems—nervous, immune, digestive, hormonal—work together, and we're still trying to figure out exactly how all the pieces fit together.

If the intestines work with the brain to control health, what does that have to do with CBD? Researchers in 2011 looked at this very connection between the nervous system and the immune system. Their study, [35] which used mice

---

34 Marilia Carabotti,a Annunziata Scirocco,a Maria Antonietta Maselli,b and Carola Severia, *Annals of Gastroenterology.* 2015 Apr-Jun; 28(2): 203–209. "The gut-brain axis: interactions between enteric microbiota, central and enteric nervous systems."

35 De Filippis D, Esposito G, Cirillo C, Cipriano M, De Winter BY, Scuderi C, Sarnelli G, Cuomo R, Steardo L, De Man JG, Iuvone T., "Cannabidiol reduces intestinal inflammation through the control of neuroimmune axis," *PLOS One,* 2011;6(12) EPUB 2011 Dec 6.

models and human tissue biopsies, showed that CBD reduced inflammation and intestinal damage without side effects among individuals with intestinal inflammation, inflammatory bowel disease, and ulcerative colitis.

ARTHRITIS AND TOPICAL CBD

CBD can be absorbed through the skin, and the brand I carry in my clinic recently released a topical CBD product, which is offered as part of our massage treatments. Certain patients who suffer from arthritis, and other inflammatory issues like joint pain and tendonitis, have walked out of their massages with much less pain due to topical CBD. In many cases, their pain was gone entirely.

A July 2016 study published in the *European Journal of Pain*[36] looked at the effects of topical CBD on rats with arthritis and other behaviors, such as withdrawing their paw due to pain. Conventional medical treatments for arthritis often have side effects such as internal bleeding. Researchers were interested in the way topical CBD could affect pain and inflammation without side effects.

One of the problems with CBD is that it doesn't mix well with water. This can make it difficult for the body to absorb when taken by mouth. (We discussed the specific types of CBD products on the market in Chapter 6.) The appeal of

36 D.C. Hammell, L.P. Zhang, F. Ma, S.M. Abshire, S.L. McIlwrath, A.L. Stinchcomb, and K.N. Westlund, "Transdermal cannabidiol reduces inflammation and pain-related behaviours in a rat model of arthritis," *European Journal of Pain,* 2016 Jul: 20(6): 936-948.

the topical CBD I use at my clinic is that it is a full-spectrum hemp product with an aloe vera base, which allows it to be absorbed into the skin much better than just water or oil alone. This topical is also infused with essential oils that help it penetrate the skin and potentiate the effects of the CBD. This is an excellent option for those suffering from arthritis because they can rub it right on the area where they have the pain and it can be applied as needed.

This particular study concludes the topical treatment did not show any evidence of side effects while also having long-lasting benefits. The researchers maintain topical (and transdermal) CBD has the potential to be an effective treatment for arthritis and other debilitating diseases.

REAL-LIFE EXAMPLES

One day, Tonya, who is on my clinic staff, accidentally banged her hand on an open drawer. Her hand instantly bruised and swelled.

She asked me, "Do you think that the topical CBD would help?"

I hadn't thought of it being used for something like that, but it seemed like a good idea.

"Yes, rub some of it on the sore area," I said.

That's what she did. About 45 minutes later, Tonya caught my attention between patients and showed me her hand.

The bruising was completely gone and the swelling had returned to normal. She told me that it felt like nothing ever happened to her hand. Not everybody will get such dramatic results as Tonya but it shows the fast-acting benefits of the topical CBD. Tonya talked about this incident for days and now tells this story to all our patients who want to know about the product.

The topical CBD also has worked wonders for Dr. Derrick DeSilva, who is a CBD expert and world-renowned physician. Dr. DeSilva is past president of the American Nutraceutical Association and a member of the teaching faculty at JFK Medical Center in Edison, NJ. At a conference, I heard him describe how he used to experience a tremendous amount of pain in his feet after he played tennis. He began to rub topical CBD on his feet to help ease discomfort from his plantar fasciitis and his pain completely disappeared.

I recommend CBD to my patients for numerous ailments but arthritis is one of the most common. One of my female patients is a retired school teacher. She wished she could be more active but was severely limited because of her arthritis. She also took care of her elderly mother, which added stress. I recommended CBD, and when she arrived for her regular adjustment four weeks later, she was ecstatic about how much the product helped.

She felt physically better and was able to return to exercising. She also felt less stress and anxiety, which made it easier to take care of her mother. She continued to take the CBD but ran out about a week before she was scheduled to come into the clinic for her next adjustment. She immediately recognized how much the CBD had been helping because the arthritic pain had returned and she had to come back and buy more.

SKIN IRRITATION AND INFLAMMATION

If you've ever had hives or poison ivy, you know that allergic reactions can be horrible. Even allergic reactions to food can lead to itchy, irritated skin rashes. People also can suffer from chronic inflammation, psoriasis, or eczema.

A June 2018 study published in *The Journal of Pharmacology and Experimental Therapeutics*[37] examined the cellular immune system response triggered during allergic reactions and how the anti-inflammatory properties of CBD affected those reactions. The researchers found CBD was very helpful without causing damage to cells.

Skin irritation and inflammation is another ailment that could respond well to the topical form of CBD. This isn't true for every type of inflammation. For individuals who have a systematic or autoimmune problem, oral treatment is better because it will get into all of the cells in your body while topical CBD is absorbed locally, for the most part.

37 Petrosino S, Verde R, Vaia M, Allara M, Iuvone T, DiMarzo V, "Anti-inflammatory Properties of Cannabidiol, a Nonpsychotropic Cannabinoid, in Experimental Allergic Contact Dermatitis," *Journal of Pharmacology and Experimental Therapy,* 2018 Jun; 365(3): 652-663 EPUB 2018 Apr 9.

The good news is oral and topical CBD can be used together for maximum impact.

Even if allergies, eczema, or skin irritations are not always major afflictions, these results are still significant. I've suffered from poison ivy in the past and would have loved to find relief. I'm sure anyone who suffers from allergic reactions feels the same way, and studies show CBD can be effective in treating multiple forms of inflammation.

Unfortunately, CBD has not been tested on all the different kinds of inflammation, and we could wait a very long time for that to happen. But I've witnessed and learned enough to know that if I were suffering from inflammation of any kind, I would certainly start by treating it with CBD.

THE VALLEY OF PAIN

Consider the experience of Susan Gundy:

"I am 71 years old, and I have been on quite a journey through the valley of pain. [My] suicidal thoughts got so strong I grew terrified I might eventually give in. Every morning, I woke up faced with such debilitating pain I just wanted to sleep. I had to stop and pray so many times throughout this journey for the strength not to give in. This is my story.

"In 2012, I suffered four strokes, which left me unable to use one side of my body. Not only was I forced to retire but for the next two years, I had minimal movement. I worked extremely hard with my physical therapists to rehabilitate my body so I could be mobile once again, but my arthritis and bad knees only got worse over time. After undergoing both a hip and shoulder replacement, the pain got so bad it felt like my body was slowly dying.

"In January 2015, I moved into a new house but there was very little insulation and it was freezing cold in the winter. When the ceiling collapsed during a failed remodeling project, I was confined to one room with a space heater for an entire month. The cold and my inability to move caused the inflammation in my body to spread from my jaw down to my feet. The pain was so severe I had to take Aleve and Tylenol regularly, but it wasn't enough.

"In April of that same year, I was diagnosed with uterine cancer, and in August, I had to have a total hysterectomy. Doctors prescribed hydrocodone to help manage the pain.

"The following year, I tore both menisci (lateral and medial) and pulled a muscle in the back of my right knee. I could not put any weight on my right leg and had to undergo arthroscopic surgery to repair the damage. While receiving regular shots in my knee to alleviate the pain, I was prescribed heavy doses of oxycodone, which ruined my digestive system.

"In 2017, my son, who worked with a high-quality health and wellness company, recommended one of the company's CBD products and gave me a bottle of the oil for Mother's

Day. I started taking the supplement and within three days, the pain began to subside but it was still there. I called my son and he suggested that I take it twice a day. I ordered some more and did what he said. That's when something amazing happened—the pain went away.

"Since October 2017, I have not taken any NSAIDs, opioids, or even any Tylenol. I no longer receive any shots in my knee. I am back to taking only one dose of CBD per day unless I plan on doing some heavy work or lots of walking and then I'll take two. I feel better than I have in years! I am so grateful that this product has allowed me to move again and gave me back my independence. Something as simple as being able to get in and out of a chair without feeling pain is a blessing. It makes me realize how grateful I am to have my life back."

THE BODY CAN HEAL ITSELF

This is how Jasper Ray describes his experience:

"In 1993, I suffered from debilitating pain and nausea with intermittent vomiting. Exploratory surgery revealed a bowel obstruction. Over the next 25 years, I underwent a series of tests with no further improvement. The ongoing diagnosis was irritable bowel syndrome (IBS), and the doctors recommended medical marijuana. That helped with the symptoms and allowed me to eat. Without it, I struggled to maintain even a reasonably healthy weight. It has gotten worse as I've gotten older. In June, my condition progressed to the point where I needed to apply for disability.

"At the beginning of September 2018, I received a text from a friend in Illinois telling me about the benefits of CBD. I told her I tried two different kinds of CBD oil and that the medical marijuana was better than both. But I decided to try the brand she recommended, which was a full-spectrum hemp oil CBD, and it proved to be one of the best decisions I've ever made. By the third day, I could tell the product was helping my gut heal and wasn't just treating the symptoms. I began to have an appetite that I had never had before in my life. Rather than being nauseous and hungry, I was just hungry. For me, that was a terrific thing!

"I was 5'8" and weighed 126 pounds when I started taking the CBD and have since gained 10 much-needed pounds. I stopped taking the medical marijuana. I can feel my body healing itself while relieving my chronic pain and nausea. I am no longer interested in receiving disability and look forward to being able to work every day. This product changed my life, and I couldn't be more thankful."

CHAPTER ELEVEN

PEACE OF MIND FOR PEOPLE WITH EPILEPSY

Few things are as frightening as watching a friend or loved one experience an epileptic seizure. It's also dangerous for the person involved because often seizures come without warning. While suffering a seizure, people can fall, hit their head, or break bones. In severe cases, they might vomit or lose control of their bowels or bladder. Even normal, everyday things like driving or swimming can be perilous for someone who suffers from epilepsy.

Individuals who suffer from epilepsy worry about the actual seizure and live in fear of what might trigger that seizure. Loud noises, bright lights, migraine headaches, alcohol, stress, and even hormones have been known to trigger seizures.

Pharmaceutical drugs are widely prescribed, and there are a number that help to prevent seizures, but unfortunately, all of them have significant side effects, including sleepiness, dizziness, nausea, weight gain, depression, confusion, skin problems, and a lack of appetite. Some patients experience difficulty thinking and even speaking in more extreme cases. It's for those reasons alone that CBD is such an appealing option for the treatment of epilepsy and seizures.

WHAT DOES THE SCIENCE TELL US?

Cannabis has been used for centuries to treat seizure disorders but that ended when cannabis was made illegal. In *The Scientist*, a 2015 documentary about cannabis, Dr. Raphael Mechoulam tells the story of a fifteenth century Arab leader who suffered from epilepsy and was treated with cannabis to control the condition for the remainder of his life. Modern research has helped to prove what many ancient civilizations already knew.

A December 2017 study[38] looked at two different types of childhood epileptic seizure conditions: Dravet Syndrome and Lennox-Gastaut Syndrome. Researchers conducted two separate double-blind studies that showed there was a dramatic improvement in the group treated with CBD when compared to the group given a placebo. One study showed a 39 percent reduction in seizure frequency compared to only a 13 percent reduction in the placebo group. In the second study, there was a 44 percent reduction in the CBD group compared to a 22 percent reduction in the placebo group. A third study attempted to look at dosage.

38 Perucca, Emilio., "Cannabinoids in the Treatment of Epilepsy: Hard Evidence at Last?" *Journal of Epilepsy Research*, 2017 Dec; 7(2): 61-76.

The group given 20 milligrams of CBD experienced a 42 percent reduction in seizure frequency while those only getting 10 milligrams experienced a 37 percent decrease.

As with most of the studies I cite throughout this book, these findings were not an isolated incident. In July of 2018, a systematic review of multiple observational studies of CBD in the treatment of epilepsy was published in the *Journal of Neurology, Neurosurgery and Psychiatry*[39]. The results clearly showed CBD reduced seizure frequency and improved the quality of life of patients suffering from epilepsy.

As a chiropractor, I am not licensed to prescribe drugs, and patients should always discuss medications with their medical doctor. I also am not licensed to give people information about discontinuing drugs, so anyone reading this book should always consult with their healthcare provider or medical doctor about any decision to discontinue any medication that has been recommended for their conditions.

There are conditions that require drugs, and epilepsy is a serious condition, but it is important to keep in mind that every drug has side effects. In my opinion, the fewer drugs that you can take, the better off you are. I'm not alone in this thinking. It's a trend. People are becoming more aware of side effects and want to reduce their overall dependency on drugs. Given the severity of epilepsy drug side effects, it

---

39 Stockings E, Zagic D, Campbell G, Weier M, Hall WD, Nielsen S, Herkes GK, Farrell M, Degenhardt L. "Evidence for cannabis and cannabinoids for epilepsy: a systematic review of controlled and observational evidence," *Journal of Neurology, Neurosurgery and Psychiatry*, 2018 Jul;89(7); 741-753 EPUB 2018 Mar 6.

seems worth trying a natural plant-based substance such as CBD, which has none.

THE DANGER OF PHARMACEUTICALS

Patients often ask me if they have to worry about interactions between CBD and other medications they may be taking. But you don't have to choose between a natural remedy such as CBD or the pharmaceutical approach. Let's look at clobazam, which is one of the most popular pharmaceuticals used to treat seizures caused by Lennox-Gastaut Syndrome. The drug can cause paranoid or suicidal ideation while impairing memory and coordination.

In June 2015, *Epilepsia* published a study[40] that showed CBD to be a safe and effective treatment for refractory epilepsy and patients taking clobazam. Researchers said it was important to monitor clobazam levels but that it was nonetheless safe to combine the two.

Even though CBD can be taken in conjunction with prescription medication, what I find revealing about the approach to this particular study is that the researchers came at it from the premise that people absolutely have to take the seizure medication. That doesn't have to be the situation for all patients. I find a growing trend among medical doctors in my area who are starting to use CBD with their patients for the treatment of various conditions, and I expect

40 Geffrey, Alexandra L., Pollack, Sarah F., Bruno, Patricia L., Thiele, Elizabeth A., "Drug-drug interaction between clobazam and cannabidiol in children with refractory epilepsy," *Epilepsia*, Volume 56, Issue 8.

this trend to dramatically increase as more people seek out natural alternatives and more research on natural products shows positive results.

THE FUTURE OF CBD DRUGS

In June 2018, Epidiolex[41] became the first cannabidiol-derived drug to treat two rare but severe forms of epilepsy to be approved by the US Food and Drug Administration (FDA). It is a prescription pharmaceutical formulation of highly purified, plant-derived cannabidiol (CBD), a cannabinoid lacking the high associated with marijuana and the first in a new category of antiepileptic drugs.

Epidiolex is made from a CBD isolate so it's not a full-spectrum hemp oil. That means that it doesn't have the combined potency of the hundreds of chemicals and cannabinoids working together, which is referred to as the entourage effect. An isolate is merely one compound.

Studies have shown[42] that when the various types of cannabinoids are administered together, the compounds work synergistically. In other words, they work better together. I recommend my patients use full-spectrum hemp oil and not an isolate. It should be no surprise that the whole is greater than the sum of the parts. God created this wonder-

41 Brodwin, Eric., "The Drug maker behind the first FDA-approved medication derived from marijuana has revealed how much it'll cost," *Business Insider,* August 8, 2018.
42 Calignano A., La Rana G., Giuffrida A., Piomelli, D., "Control of pain initiation by endogenous cannabinoids," *Nature,* 1998 Jul 16;394(6690); 277-81.

ful plant with a whole bunch of beneficial cannabinoids, so why not use it as intended?

I can only speculate why they would use an isolate for this particular drug, but companies are attracted to isolates since you can patent a synthetic version of a natural product. It's common for manufacturers to isolate one component and create a synthetic version, which also allows them to better control their product. There is some variability with natural hemp, depending on where it was grown, how much sun it received, whether it was organic, and what nutrients were in the ground. When using an isolate, companies can guarantee control and produce a product that can be consistently replicated.

Epidiolex appears not to have the same dangerous side effects as the other, more dangerous drugs used to treat seizures but side effects aren't the only downfall of modern-day pharmaceuticals. Once a drug company has a patent and FDA approval, it has the exclusive rights to that drug. They can then charge pretty much whatever the market dictates since other companies won't be able to manufacture that drug for a certain period of time.

According to a *Business Insider* article by Eric Brodwin from August 8, 2018, GW Pharmaceuticals announced that Epidiolex would cost roughly $32,500 per year for a prescription, which is an enormous amount of money and just goes to show the level of greed in the pharmaceutical industry. By comparison, the CBD product I use at my clinic would cost only $1,500 per year, a savings of $31,000.

SUPPLEMENTS AND THE FDA

FDA regulation has tremendous associated costs, and generally products are pursued only if they have a high return on investment.

The FDA doesn't regulate vitamins or supplements, which is both good and bad. It means there isn't as much oversight with supplements and you have to be careful about their origins. You need to understand the manufacturer's testing and quality control measures, making sure their products are verified by an outside lab. You want to know that the product contains the advertised active ingredient and doesn't contain impurities. It should meet label requirements, including potency and effectiveness. It's not required but a good company will do these things, even if it costs more for them to produce and for the consumer to buy.

CBD WORKS FOR EPILEPSY

Here is what Janet Fastuca says about CBD:

"It all started September 2017 when I was at the Notre Dame vs. Georgia football game. I was standing in line, waiting to get in, when I began to feel nauseous. Granted, I had been tailgating all day and had a couple of drinks, but this was different. Something wasn't right. I felt dizzy and was about to pass out, so I sat down.

"The paramedics took me into the stadium where they tested my blood sugar. I was there for about a half-hour when I started to vomit. I thought I might be suffering from food poisoning because we had been eating food that was out all day, but when I started to get sick again, the paramedics took me to the emergency room.

"I wasn't there long. They monitored me, gave me some medication to stop the vomiting, and sent me home without a diagnosis. I went on my merry way thinking that was it.

"It happened again two weeks before Christmas. My husband and I were out to dinner with friends when I started to get that same nauseous feeling. I passed out this time but my husband caught me, so I wasn't hurt during the fall. When I woke up, I still felt nauseous. My husband took me home. I vomited for several hours. The next day, I was exhausted and couldn't eat. I was able to get some food down on the second day, but I had absolutely no energy.

"My first appointment was with a neurologist. When they took my blood pressure, the nurse was concerned. 'Are you about to pass out?'

"'No, I feel fine,' I told her.

"I always had low blood pressure so I wasn't alarmed, but I took her advice and went to see the cardiologist. He verified that I had low blood pressure but he didn't seem concerned either. He sent me home and told me to 'enjoy my salt.' That was it.

"I went to see an ear, nose, and throat specialist and made a lot of calls, trying to figure out what the problem was, but given my high insurance deductible, I didn't want to go overboard.

"On March 5, 2018, I was driving home after a night with my girlfriends when I felt tired. My husband was out of town, but when I got home, I called him and told him I didn't feel well so I was going to bed early. Around 11:30 p.m., I woke up feeling nauseous so I went to the bathroom, assumed the position, and then passed out. I woke up in a puddle of vomit. I had also hit my head and twisted my neck. I was disoriented and started to gag but was able to regroup, clean up, and go back to bed. At 2:30 a.m., I woke up again, went to the bathroom, and the same thing happened. This is bad. Something is not right

"I went back to the doctor. I had an MRI and a slew of different tests. The final test was an EEG. My doctor said that I suffered from epileptic seizures, which is unusual because adults don't typically first experience seizures later in life. I did my research and learned that one of the causes of seizures is migraines.

"I believe in a natural and holistic approach to medicine. I don't like to take prescription drugs if I don't have to but I will if I need to so when the doctor prescribed me medication to make the seizures stop, I asked if there was anything else I could do. I just started to learn about CBD during my research and brought it up to her, but she told me that I couldn't take the CBD by itself and suggested I take it along with the prescription. I reluctantly filled the prescription and brought it home but grew concerned when I saw all the potential side effects.

"I decided to take only the CBD and no prescription medications. I did my research, consulted with the people at a health food store, and they got me started on CBD in pill form. It was oil in a capsule. They told me if I felt a seizure coming on, to bite down and let the oil get into my system which could stop a seizure from even happening. I was able to put that to the test a few weeks later when I was on a weekend trip with friends to Chicago. When we were out at dinner, I started to feel nauseous, so I bit down on the pill. I had no idea what would happen next and I didn't want to ruin their night, so I asked that they take me back to the house where I was staying. As soon as we got in the car, I closed my eyes, said a prayer, and went to sleep. When we arrived at the house 45 minutes later, the nausea was gone.

"That was my first experience with CBD and I knew that it was the real deal. I wanted to get involved with doctors who believed in CBD. I continued to do my research, and out of the five doctors I've seen, two have believed in me and agreed to work with me. The most recent is Dr. Mark Lindholm. He had been researching CBD for the past year because of his own situation. I had been a patient of his for a long time and I trusted him, so I purchased the product he recommended and tried it for a month. I did exactly what I was told to do and have been seizure free for six months. There are times I can feel a bout of nausea coming on and that's when I take a little extra under my tongue. Within 20 minutes, that nausea is gone.

"I still keep that first prescription I received from my doctor in the medicine cabinet as a reminder. CBD has been a blessing for me and for my husband, who is a former college football player and has been taking the CBD as an alternative to prescription drugs for his aches and pains. And it's not just us. There are thousands of people out there who have stories just as remarkable."

CHAPTER TWELVE

CAN WE SLOW THE SPREAD OF DEMENTIA?

One of my dearest relatives, and a constant role model for me, suffers from dementia. He never went to college, but before the dementia he had the kind of wisdom that comes from experience. He was a farmer, but like many family farmers, he also always worked another job to make ends meet. During planting and harvesting season, he'd be out in the fields working late into the night. Even though he was busy, he was the first to help someone in need. I loved to spend time with him and just talk, even though his hearing started to go a few years ago and he had trouble tracking conversations.

One day not long before writing this book, we were playing cards. This was a favorite pastime of ours over the years, and we often had the best conversations while playing. When I was young, he even taught me how to play cribbage. It's a somewhat complicated game but we played it together for decades. On this particular day, he couldn't remember the rules, and I had to explain it to him—the very game he had taught me to play many years earlier. That was a sobering moment for me. I realized he wasn't just suffering from hearing problems. We later learned that he was suffering from dementia.

Dementia is a scary thing. Anyone who has watched a loved one suffer from dementia understands this. Your loved one is still there, but their essence slowly disappears. Luckily, my dear relative's symptoms remain relatively mild and we were able to get him into a great holistic clinic which has a "memory rescue program" geared toward helping dementia. He started treatment and we are expecting, hoping, and praying for some improvement in his condition. In addition to other holistic approaches, I got him to try CBD, and the nutritionist we worked with as part of the memory rescue program recommended that he continue using it.

Treatment for dementia is typically aimed at treating the symptoms. We're hoping to treat the cause.

CBD AND ALZHEIMER'S

Alzheimer's disease begins with short-term memory loss, particularly the ability to learn and communicate. In the moderate stage, these issues start to impact everyday life, and by the later stage, there are severe impairments in the patient's ability to speak and recognize people. Some people in the later stages of Alzheimer's require 24-hour care.

Unfortunately, no mainstream treatments can stop or reverse Alzheimer's. There are only four approved drugs to treat it, and they all have side effects that include nausea, vomiting, diarrhea, weight loss, fatigue, dizziness, and even hallucinations. Even though experts acknowledge more research needs to be done on CBD and its potential to treat dementia, the results are promising.

A February 2017 study published in *Frontiers in Pharmacology*[43] reviewed five different CBD studies related to Alzheimer's. In one of the studies, three-month-old mice were injected daily with a dose of CBD for one week and then injected three times per week for the following two weeks. Researchers then assessed the special learning capabilities of the mice using a device called the Morris Water Maze, which is a navigation test commonly used with rodents to study learning and memory. The mouse is placed in a circular pool. It must escape the water and find a platform using a series of various cues. The mouse either remembers the movements, relies on visual cues, or implements a special strategy. When the results were in, CBD was shown to reverse and prevent the development of cognitive deficits in Alzheimer's rodent models while also being "perfectly placed to treat a number of pathologies typically found in Alzheimer's."

Researchers also studied possible preventative treatment in mice. The mice were treated for eight months with CBD to study the long-term effect of CBD before they showed

43 Watt, Georgia., Karl, Tim., "In vivo Evidence of Therapeutic Properties of Cannabidiol (CBD) for Alzheimer's Disease," *Frontiers in Pharmacology,* 2017; 8:20.

symptoms of Alzheimer's. Researchers determined treating mice with CBD was able to "prevent the development of social recognition memory deficits without affecting anxiety domains" in mice with Alzheimer's genes. This bears repeating: The Frontiers in Pharmacology Studies showed reversal of Alzheimer's symptoms and prevention of the development of Alzheimer's Disease!

According to the Alzheimer's Association, 5.7 million Americans are living with the disease. By 2050, this number is projected to rise to nearly 14 million. One in three seniors in America dies with Alzheimer's or another type of dementia, and Alzheimer's kills more than breast cancer and prostate cancer combined. That is an enormous amount of suffering and a tremendous number of patients and loved ones who would undoubtedly like to know that CBD may have the potential to prevent and reverse their symptoms[44].

THE BENEFITS OF CBD & THC TOGETHER

A previously cited study published in *Frontiers in Pharmacology* looked at the effectiveness of CBD combined with THC, showing that in some cases it could provide more therapeutic benefits than either cannabinoid alone.

In some cases, "THC alone had a detrimental effect on cognition in control mice, highlighting the need to be cautious when considering THC as therapeutic," the study said. "However, control mice treated with a CBD-THC

44 Alzheimer's Association Website, www.alz.org/alzheimers-dementia/facts-figures.

combination did not show any cognitive deficits, suggesting that CBD may be able to antagonize the detrimental effects of THC."

In other words, CBD seems to be more effective and safer than THC and the addition of CBD to THC seems to reduce the downsides of THC. THC is the chemical that makes people high from marijuana.

The studies provide proof of principle for the therapeutic benefits of CBD and possible CBD-THC combinations. More research is required, especially on older mice because many of the studies were conducted on younger mice and Alzheimer's usually emerges later in life.

Nevertheless, the studies discussed here provide promising preliminary data and the translation of this preclinical work to the clinical setting could be realized relatively quickly: CBD is readily available, appears to have limited side effects, and is safe for human use.

A recent study[45], "Neurological Aspects of Medical Use of Cannabidiol," looked specifically at all of the preclinical and clinical findings related to CBD as the sole treatment of neurological and neuropsychiatric disorders. The findings didn't just relate to Alzheimer's or one type of dementia. They also included laboratory and clinical studies on the potential role of CBD in treatment for Parkinson's,

45 Mannucci C, Navarra M, Calapai F, Spagnolo EV, Busardò FP, Cas RD, Ippolito FM, Calapai G., "Neurological Aspects of Medical Use of Cannabidiol," *CNS & Neurological Disorders Drug Targets,* 2017; 16(5);541-553.

Alzheimer's, multiple sclerosis, Huntington's disease, ALS, and cerebral ischemia.

While there are only a few human studies, the preclinical evidence suggests CBD benefits patients with Alzheimer's, Parkinson's disease, and multiple sclerosis.

WHY IS CBD EFFECTIVE?

Researchers and medical professionals have been at an impasse when it comes to treating Alzheimer's. A 2014 study in *Frontiers in Pharmacology*[46] cited the limited effectiveness of current therapies and highlighted the need for more research efforts devoted to developing new products for preventing or delaying the disease. Alzheimer's is a unique disease in that the early stages of the neurodegenerative process and symptomatic stages may take decades to progress but the progress accelerates at a certain point. That's why researchers are looking for ways to treat the disease at the beginning stages. Even four years ago, researchers pointed out how "targeting the endogenous cannabinoid system has emerged as a potential therapeutic approach to treat" Alzheimer's.

Diving deeper, the 2014 study suggests: "Several findings indicate that the activation of both CB_1 and CB_2 receptors by natural or synthetic agonists, at non-psychoactive doses, have beneficial effects in Alzheimer's experimental models

46 Aso, Ester., Ferrer, Isidre., "Cannabinoids for treatment of Alzheimer's disease: moving toward the clinic," *Frontiers in Pharmacology.* 2014; 5:37.

by reducing the harmful β-amyloid peptide action and tau phosphorylation, as well as by promoting the brain's intrinsic repair mechanisms. Moreover, endocannabinoid signaling has been demonstrated to modulate numerous concomitant pathological processes, including neuroinflammation, excitotoxicity, mitochondrial dysfunction, and oxidative stress."

In other words, using CBD actually reduced the cause of Alzheimer's (the formation of amyloid plaques) and improved the patient's ability to heal. It also simultaneously reduced other problems, including brain inflammation, toxicity, cellular energy dysfunction, and oxidative stress known to injure the brain.

The study also points out something we've seen in previous studies, which is that neuronal damage can increase the production of endocannabinoids, which is the body's natural way to fight back against disease and infection. This is exactly what happens in pancreatic cancer cells. What this means is that when there is a problem, the body seems to naturally increase the receptors to which CBD binds or is attracted and ramps up the possibility of the CBD working better.

The body seems to know that it needs more activation of the endocannabinoid system. However, if you are not supplementing your body with a high-quality hemp or CBD product, it is like having more locks without the keys.

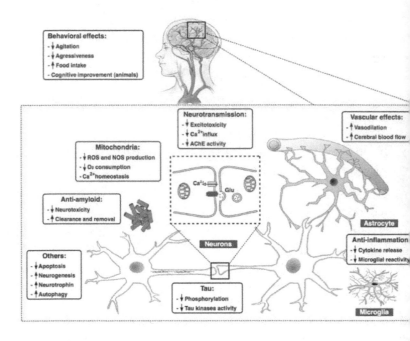

Summary of the main findings demonstrating beneficial effects of cannabinoid compounds in AD models. Cannabinoids may target in parallel several processes that play key roles in AD, including Aβ and tau aberrant processing, chronic inflammatory responses, excitotoxicity, mitochondrial dysfunction, and oxidative stress, among others. Clinical data also reveal an improvement in behavioral in patients with AD after treatment with cannabinoids.

Source: Aso, Ester., Ferrer, Isidre., "Cannabinoids for treatment of Alzheimer's disease: moving toward the clinic," Frontiers in Pharmacology, 2014; 5:37

The possible neuroprotective effects of CBD make it a promising Alzheimer's treatment. One study from the

Journal of Neurochemistry[47] looked specifically at the oxidative stress levels of in vitro-cultured rat cells. Researchers discovered that when they pretreated these cells with CBD, there was significant increase in cell survival compared to cells not treated with CBD.

Beta-amyloids are protein fragments in the brain that are expelled in healthy people but can damage nerve cells in people with Alzheimer's. Scientists at Stanford University School of Medicine have shown that the protein fragments in beta-amyloids are one of the likely causes of Alzheimer's. They begin destroying synapses or nerve cell connections before they clump together into plaques that lead to nerve cell or brain cell death. These synapses or nerve connections are essential for storing memories and processing thoughts and emotions.

A similar mouse study[48] found CBD significantly prevented neuroinflammation (nerve swelling and damage) found in Alzheimer's.

"The results of the present study confirm in vivo anti-inflammatory actions of CBD, emphasizing the importance of this compound as a novel promising pharmacological tool capable of attenuating A-beta evoked neuroinflammatory responses," researchers concluded.

47 Iuvone T, Esposito G, Esposito R, Santamaria R, Di Rosa M, Izzo AA., "Neuroprotective effect of cannabidiol, a non-psychoactive component from Cannabis sativa, on beta-amyloid-induced toxicity in PC12 cells," *Journal of Neurochemistry*, 2004 Ap;89(1); 134-41.

48 Esposito G, Scuderi C, Savani C, Steardo L Jr, De Filippis D, Cottone P, Iuvone T, Cuomo V, Steardo L., "Cannabidiol in vivo blunts beta-amyloid induced neuroinflammation by suppressing IL-1beta and iNOS expression," *British Journal of Pharmacology*, 2007 Aug; 151(8): 1272-9 EPUB 2007 Jan 25.

HOW MUCH LONGER CAN WE WAIT?

Dementia affected an estimated 5.7 million Americans in 2018, according to the Alzheimer's Association, with Alzheimer's projected to impact 14 million people by the year 2050[49].

The management and treatment of that many people, combined with the fact we don't really have good treatment options, poses an enormous healthcare concern. We need more CBD research to address this oncoming wave.

REBOOTING FROM A TRAUMATIC BRAIN INJURY

Here is the story of Krystin Rowe:

"In 2005, I suffered a traumatic brain injury. I spent the next 18 months trying to 'reboot,' but I experienced a series of losses and setbacks.

"For the first two months, I had difficulty walking and standing. It took a lot of thought and I moved very slowly. I experienced double vision and would see two complete pictures. Light, sound, smell, and speed were all intensified beyond my level of comfort. I suffered from aphasia, which is the inability to say what I was thinking. I had difficulty holding small items. I suffered amnesia—if I hadn't seen someone within 48 hours, I had no idea who they were. I

49 *Alzheimer's Association Website, www.alz.org/alzheimers-dementia/facts-figures.

cried for no reason at all. I suffered from horrible headaches and complete numbness on the right side of my face where the injury occurred. I could no longer play the piano as I had before the TBI. At times my voice wavered and at other times it felt like I didn't have a voice. That could last for days at a time. My family struggled to interpret what I was trying to say and basic communication was difficult.

"My boss recommended I try full-spectrum hemp derived CBD oil. From the very first time I used it, the difference was obvious. By the second day, I felt more awake and focused. I wasn't walking around like a zombie. I felt awesome!

"Today, I can focus and stay alert all day without suffering from any headaches. I think that adding the topical CBD to the base of my neck has really helped with that as well. I sleep well at night. I speak with a strong voice. I can articulate what I want to say. I remember the names of people from my past and those who I recently met. It feels like I've regained access to those memories that I feared were lost forever—my school days, time spent with my grandparents, my wedding, the birth of my children and my grandchildren. I feel like I am whole again. I have experienced so many different benefits from CBD. Here are just a few examples:

- After the accident, my left eye became cloudy and I began to lose my vision. I panicked at first but it has gotten clearer each day. In fact, I see rather well today for a person who has been nearsighted since first grade.

- The scars from various surgeries would create a pinching type of pain but that pain has begun to subside.

- I had experienced horrible pain in my left arm after surgery to remove a tumor and about one-third of my muscle in the area back in 2006. Two years ago, the tumor began to grow back but has since stopped in its tracks.

- I have found tremendous benefits from the topical CBD I apply to my surgery sites daily. I've seen improvement but don't believe that the area is fully healed yet.

- Back in 1990, I broke my hip and dislocated my pelvis. Although the hip healed pretty well, the pelvis issue was not diagnosed for almost a year until my ability to walk became severely impaired. The muscle atrophied, and I underwent therapy to stretch it out again. It hasn't bothered me since, but the CBD awakened the area and I felt some pain as the old injury was repaired.

- I am not allowed to have any vaccinations due to a compromised immune system from leukemia. However, I noticed last week that, as everyone in my office was experiencing the autumn cough from pollen (which has been a real problem for me my whole life), I breathed freely and didn't cough. In fact, I haven't even taken my asthma inhaler to work with me in months. I just keep realizing more and more great ways I feel healed.

"I tell myself that the CBD is searching for all needed repairs and is tackling them one by one. I have been comfortable taking a little extra if needed one day and backing off entirely for a day or two if I feel it is 'healing me too quickly.'

"I recently began experimenting with putting a small bit of topical on some moles and tags to see if they would disappear. So far, I have seen some of the areas lighten in color, and I feel very optimistic.

"CBD has been a life changer for me. Since I was never a drinker, smoker, or recreational drug taker, I have never wanted to take a product that would make me feel weird or heady like some of my prescriptions have left me feeling. The CBD has never given me any strange feeling. I genuinely believe that CBD has restored my health and well-being and is continuing to do so."

CHAPTER THIRTEEN

CBD AND YOUR HEART

Everyone understands a heart attack, but people aren't sure what to make of the term "heart disease."

It's not just one disease; it's an entire class of diseases that involve the heart and blood vessels. That includes everything from coronary artery disease, angina, heart attack, stroke, heart failure, and high blood pressure. Heart disease is the number one cause of death for both men and women, according to the Centers for Disease Control and Prevention (CDC), a federal agency under the Department of Health and Human Services that is headquartered in Atlanta, Georgia.

HOW CAN CBD HELP?

We already know CBD reduces inflammation. Since inflammation is at the root of the cause of heart disease, it's no surprise CBD can be beneficial.

A 2013 study in the *British Journal of Clinical Pharmacology*[50] found that CBD improves blood flow and protects against heart damage caused by high sugar levels in animals with type 2 diabetes. Proper blood flow is essential so the body can deliver oxygen and other nutrients while removing waste products. What makes heart disease so dangerous is the closing off of the arteries, which limits blood flow. Sometimes that can be caused by plaques or other blockages in the arteries, but sometimes it's due to the tightening of blood vessels that, either independently or along with blockages, impede blood flow.

When there is a temporary lack of blood flow to the heart or brain, it can cause inflammation, and heart or brain damage. CBD treatment protects against this, studies show. In other words, it opens blood vessels, assists blood flow, and protects against damage. The *British Journal of Pharmacology* [38] also showed that it can protect your heart by reducing damage caused by a heart attack.

AN OUNCE OF PREVENTION

If someone who had CBD in their system suffered a heart attack, they could have a smaller chance of dying and experience less damage to the heart than someone without CBD. Also, if someone having a heart attack was given CBD, it could reduce damage to the heart.

50 Stanley, Christopher P., Hind, William H., O'Sullivan, Saoirse E., "Is the cardiovascular system a therapeutic target for cannabidiol?" *British Journal of Pharmacology,* 2013 Feb; 75(2): 313-322.

These findings come from a study in the *British Journal of Pharmacology*[51] that gave rats CBD and induced heart attacks. Researchers looked at what happened when the blood flow returned to their hearts. They studied heartbeats and later removed the hearts to inspect damage to the tissue. The results were amazing: CBD significantly reduced the cardiac problems. In addition, they found rats given CBD (only after restricting the blood flow to the heart, and not before) also experienced less damage.

PROMISING RESULTS IN HUMANS

CBD and its impact on heart disease is an area that needs more research. Given the severity of heart disease and the fact that someone dies from a heart attack every 38 seconds, further work is needed to support these findings, establish protocols, and confirm whether this also happens in humans.

In the meantime, a June 2017 randomized, placebo-controlled, double-blind, crossover study[52] attempted to look at how a single dose of CBD could reduce blood pressure. Nine healthy male volunteers were given either 600 mg of CBD or a placebo. Since it was double-blind, neither the

51 Walsh, SK., Hepburn CY., Kane KA., Wainwright CL., "Acute administration of cannabidiol in vivo suppresses ischaemia-induced cardiac arrhythmias and reduces infarct size when given at reperfusion," *British Journal of Pharmacology,* 2010 Jul:160(5); 1234-42.
52 Jadoon, Khalid A., Tan, Gary D., O'Sullivan, Saoirse E., "A single dose of cannabidiol reduces blood pressure in healthy volunteers in a randomized crossover study," *JCI Insight,* 2017 Jun 15; 2(12).

participants nor the researchers knew who received the active ingredient.

They found CBD reduced the resting blood pressure by 6 mm of mercury. To put this in context, if you have a blood pressure of 146/86, CBD could on average bring it down to 140/80. It also reduced how much blood the heart pushed out when it was beating. They studied the subjects both at rest and when stressed, and they had the same results. The data showed that even when the heart was pumping faster, CBD lowered blood pressure.

High blood pressure is a major risk factor for developing heart disease, and this study shows CBD is significant in reducing blood pressure. What makes these findings so important, and slightly different from some of the conditions discussed in other chapters, is that up to 90 percent of heart disease is preventable. Eating healthy, exercising, avoiding tobacco, and limiting alcohol intake can help prevent it.

Imagine if you began using this safe, healthy, and effective plant-based supplement along with exercise and a healthy diet. That could greatly reduce your chance of developing heart disease.

CBD, HEART DISEASE, AND SLEEP

It's well-documented that sleep disorders such as insomnia can increase your risk of developing heart disease. Not only has CBD been shown to help individuals fall asleep and stay asleep but in my personal experience (and that of many of my patients) it helps provide a deeper sleep.

With CBD, I found myself dreaming more. I awoke more rested and with more energy. I seemed to feel better with less sleep, which I attribute to getting into that deep REM sleep. I've heard my patients tell me these same things over and over again, and most reported this after only a few days of taking the product. This is crucial because our cardio-vascular health, brains, and immune system, among other aspects of the human body require quality sleep to function optimally.

Some of the wonderful benefits of CBD don't happen immediately. Sometimes it takes a month or two to derive the full benefit of CBD for conditions like pain and inflammation. This is especially true for longstanding issues like heart health, autoimmune diseases, and chronic levels of inflammation due to colitis or joint damage from arthritis.

Some patients have a hard time following through on a treatment, medication, or lifestyle change if they don't experience an instant benefit. Many of my patients who started taking CBD for more severe conditions might have stopped taking the product, too, had they not been getting better sleep and felt more rested. That response alone was beneficial enough for them to keep taking the CBD long enough to get its full benefits.

This is important because heart disease is a silent killer. Most people don't learn they have heart disease until they have a heart attack. High blood pressure and many of the problems associated with heart disease have little to no symptoms before a life-threatening event. Since CBD has been shown to prevent these problems before patients even realize there's an issue, it can be a great benefit.

CHAPTER FOURTEEN

BOOSTING YOUR IMMUNE SYSTEM TO FIGHT INFECTIONS

Landfills attract rats, but nobody makes the mistake of thinking that rats created them. That would be backward. Rats were attracted to the landfill because there was food to eat. To think that a bacterial or viral infection causes disease or makes a person sick is also backward. First, the body has been weakened.

The chiropractic approach is to strengthen the way the body works instead of viewing microorganisms as the threat. Our aim is to boost the immune system's ability to fight off dangerous bacteria. It's more about promoting good health than it is fighting disease, which runs counter to the view of conventional medicine.

Our environment is overrun with bacteria. There isn't a surface on the face of the earth that isn't saturated with it. When people get the idea to sterilize their environment to get rid of bacteria, they are fighting a losing battle. It can't be done. The same is true about viruses. It's believed that there are one million times as many viruses in this world as there are stars in the universe. That's a considerable number, and it's impossible to fight them all.

These days, it's common practice to take antibiotics when we get an infection. Most people don't think twice about it. One of the problems with antibiotics is that they take a shotgun-style approach to infections that also kill the healthy bacteria. Some strains of bacteria have even become resistant to antibiotics because of overuse. The bacteria became stronger and learned to survive, so these antibiotics are no longer effective against them.

Nor are antibiotics effective against viruses, and we don't have many good medications for viral infections. For a long time, cannabis has been known to contain antibacterial properties, but how effective can it be in treating infections and viruses?

THE RESEARCH

Unlike antibiotics that attempt to kill bacteria, CBD works by boosting the immune system. This strengthens the body. Sometimes the traditional approach of trying to kill the infection is necessary but it overlooks the preventative aspect.

There also is evidence that CBD can suppress some T-cell

function in the immune system[53]. This isn't always a bad thing. Why would we want to suppress our immune system? Many people today suffer from autoimmune diseases, which occur when the body becomes overactive and attacks itself. A condition like rheumatoid arthritis is an autoimmune disease. In fact, many chronic diseases are thought to be autoimmune disease, and if CBD can suppress T-cell function, it could help combat these types of diseases.

In addition to boosting the immune system, CBD also has been shown to potentially have an antiviral and an antibacterial effect. Endocannabinoids indirectly activate neutrophils, which are part of white blood cells that circulate throughout the body and are often the first cells to travel to an injured or infected part of the body. They fight infection by releasing enzymes that kill microorganisms and fight both bacterial and viral infections[54].

CBD also has been shown to be effective against certain strains of MRSA, for instance. Infections such as MRSA are the type of infections that people tend to get in hospitals or other medical centers. A 2008 study in the *Journal of Natural Products*[55] studied the five main cannabinoids and learned they all acted with potency against certain strains

53 Kaplan, BL., Springs AE., Kaminski NE., "The profile of immune modulation by cannabidiol (CBD) involves deregulation of nuclear factor of activated T cells (NFAT)," *Biochemical Pharmacology,* 2008 Sep 15;76(6): 726-37 EPUB 2008 Jul 8.

54 Chouinard F, Turcotte C, Guan X, Larose MC, Poirier S, Bouchard L, Provost V, Flamand L, Grandvaux N, Flamand N., "2-Arachidonoyl-glycerol- and arachidonic acid-stimulated neutrophils release antimicrobial effectors against E. coli, S. aureus, HSV-1, and RSV," *Journal of Leukocyte Biology,* 2013 Feb; 93 (2); 267-76 EPUB 2012 Dec 12.

55 Appendino G, Gibbons S, Giana A, Pagani A, Grassi G, Stavri M, Smith E, Rahman MM., "Antibacterial cannabinoids from Cannabis sativa: a structure-activity study," *Journal of Natural Products,* 2008 Aug1 71(8): 1427-30 EPUB 2008 Aug 6.

of MRSA. This is significant because MRSA is resistant to antibiotics and can be life threatening.

ACNE BE GONE

Acne is essentially an infection of the pores in your skin, and I've had patients who experienced outstanding results when using topical CBD on acne. This is huge as other common approaches such as drugs like Accutane can have side effects. I've had other patients with rashes from fungal infections who have had similarly good results.

Unfortunately, there isn't much research in this area but some of my patients have noticed a dramatic improvement. The research we do have has shown that CBD has antibiotic and antiviral properties in addition to improving immune function.

SNAKE OIL OR MIRACLE CURE?

This is what Rebecca Gilbert Everett says about her experience with CBD:

"Back in 2016, I was in a car accident that jarred loose the six-inch plate…in my leg from a previous accident. I had to have the plate removed because it was pinching the nerves. While in the hospital, I contracted MRSA. I was put on antibiotics and steroids but the infection got into my bloodstream. My hair started to fall out. I suffered from cramps so bad that I could see my muscles tighten up and take a different shape. My ankle was swollen to the point it was almost unrecognizable, which made the neuropathy I suffered within my feet even worse. The doctors were just trying to pump me full of antibiotics until they could amputate my foot.

"In addition to my personal doctor and surgeon, I visited an internal medicine and infectious disease doctor and a dermatologist, but none of them could help me. To make things worse, my husband had been diagnosed with stage *IV* lymphoma. My anxiety level was so high I thought I was going to suffer a stroke. It was overwhelming. Most nights I lied awake in bed crying. I feared that I was going to die and reached a point where I was begging God for mercy. I was scared.

"It was during a trip to the Walgreens Minute Clinic with my husband (when we met) a nurse named Kerrie Davis, whom I knew because our kids went to school together. She took one look at me and said, 'Oh my goodness, what are you going through?' Then she saw my ankle. 'Oh, my stars, you need to come see me.'

"Kerrie invited me to attend a CBD meeting, so I decided to go. What did I have to lose? She told me to stop taking the steroids and antibiotics and start taking the CBD product she recommended every day. From the very first day, I could feel my anxiety lessen. I could finally sleep at night. I didn't experience any more charley horses, and the pain was starting to decrease. By the third night, my ankle wasn't throbbing. Within a week, the inflammation went down and I started to get some of the feeling back in my feet for the first time in years. I could get up and walk normally.

"When I returned to the doctor, he assumed the decreased swelling and the overall improvement in my condition was due to the antibiotics but I told him I stopped taking the antibiotics. I showed him the CBD product, and he called it snake oil. I couldn't help but laugh, 'Well, that snake oil is the only thing saving my foot.' Nothing that he or any of the other doctors recommended had worked. I also noticed how the CBD kept my blood sugar and diabetes in check. I believe God put things on this Earth that can heal our bodies, and CBD is one of those things. It changed my life. The rest is history. My pain and inflammation are gone. My blood pressure is normal, and I no longer suffer from any issues related to diabetes. And all I take is the CBD."

CHAPTER FIFTEEN

CAN CBD BE EFFECTIVE IN THE FIGHT AGAINST CANCER?

I remember finding out that my grandmother had cancer like it was yesterday.

You know how emotionally charged memories are precisely etched into your mind? It seems like memories from my youth are especially strong when they're tied to deep emotions. I was about eight years old, and it was my first experience watching someone whom I really loved suffer. My grandmother was in her early fifties when she was diagnosed, and it makes me furious to think how cancer stole her from me. The doctors gave her only three months to live, but they didn't really know my grandmother. She was a tough cookie. She didn't look ferocious. She couldn't have weighed more than 110 pounds, but she was a second-generation Irish immigrant and had a lot of fight in her.

She lived for three more years, but it was still incredibly painful to watch. Cancer didn't just take her; it destroyed her. Over those three years, I watched my grandmother slowly slip away. And it wasn't just cancer—it was the chemotherapy and the radiation. Thinking about that experience makes me mad, and I'm haunted by the memory of her ailing body, so I try to remember my grandmother before she was sick. I only wish that I had known about CBD then.

I know that my story isn't unique. Cancer is the second leading cause of death in the United States. The sad reality, however, is that there are only three approved treatment options routinely used for cancer in the United States—surgery, chemotherapy, and radiation. There are some newer approaches including immunotherapy, targeted or precision therapy, hormonal therapy, and stem cell transplants[56], but this is different from other countries where other treatments and approaches are used. I know many people who have traveled outside of the US in order to get access to cancer treatment options that are not available here.

THE ROADBLOCK FOR NATURAL REMEDIES

The sad truth is that there have been relatively small advances in the treatment of cancer in the US over the last 50 years. We dump a ton of money into finding a "cure," but most of that money goes toward researching treatments.

56 National Cancer Institute at the National Institutes of Health, Website: https://www. cancer.gov/about-cancer/treatment/types.

And no one has the financial incentive to spend money on developing options that use a natural product derived from a widely available plant[575859].

93 STUDIES CAN'T BE WRONG

In no way am I saying natural supplements like CBD can cure cancer but the research out there is encouraging.

"A large body of evidence shows that cannabinoids, in addition to their well-known palliative effects on some cancer-associated symptoms, can reduce tumor growth in animal models of cancer," reported a 2015 summary review of 93 different studies by researchers in Spain[60]. "They do so by modulating key cell signaling pathways involved in the control of cancer cell proliferation and survival. In addition, cannabinoids inhibit angiogenesis and cell proliferation in different types of tumors in laboratory animals."

In layman's language, the review showed cannabinoids cause your immune system to attack and kill cancer cells. Cannabinoids also were shown to inhibit angiogenesis, which is the formation of new blood vessels. That is important because cancer cells need a blood supply to rapidly divide and grow. What some of the animal studies

57 National Institutes of Health, "Yesterday, Today and Tomorrow NIH research timelines," 2007.

58 Shannon Brownlee, "Feeding the Cancer Machine," *The New York Times Op-Ed,* April 1, 2007.

59 John P. Thomas, "The Cancer Industry is Too Prosperous to Allow a Cure," *Health Impact News,* December 16, 2018.

60 Velasco G., Sanchez C., Guzman M., "Endocannabinoids and Cancer," *The Handbook of Experimental Pharmacology,* 2015; 231: 449-72.

have shown is that cannabinoids contribute to a two-fold approach that destroys the cancer cells and prevents blood vessel nutrients from reaching them.

A 2016 study published in the *European Journal of Pharmacology*[61] also showed cannabinoids have anti-cancer actions and are usually well tolerated, which means that they don't produce the toxic effects of chemotherapy. "There is considerable merit in the development of cannabinoids in anti-cancer therapy," researchers concluded.

The study also mentioned that CBD activates cancer cell death and prevents new cancer growth by inhibiting blood flow[62].

61 Javid FA, Phillips RM, Afshinjavid S, Verde R, Ligresti A, "Cannabinoid pharmacology in cancer research: A new hope for cancer patients," *European Journal of Pharmacology,* 2016 Mar 15; 775: 1-14 EPUB 2016 Feb 5.
62 Figure is from Velasco G., Sanchez C., Guzman M., "Endocannabinoids and Cancer," *The Handbook of Experimental Pharmacology*, 2015; 231: 449-72.

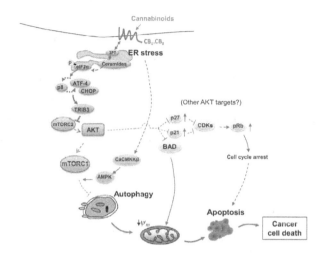

AN ALTERNATIVE TO CASTRATION

The first line of a 2015 study on prostate cancer immediately grabbed my attention: "In the early stages, prostate cancer is androgen-dependent; therefore, medical castration has shown significant results during the initial stages of this pathology." Yes, they claim that castration has shown to be beneficial in the early stages of prostate cancer. And if the term "castration" within the context of medical treatment doesn't get the attention of men out there, then I don't know what will because that's pretty scary.

That study from *Oncology Reports*[63] looked at the pre-programmed cell death of prostate cancer cells caused by endocannabinoids, the natural cannabinoids produced by your body. Natural cannabinoids bind to the same receptor sites in the body as CBD. The study takes into account evidence showing cannabinoids have a protective effect against different kinds of cancers and sought the presence of these receptors on cancer cells to show that cannabinoids may be a viable treatment for prostate cancer.

They found receptors on the prostate cancer cells but there were actually more receptors found on the cells in the later stage of the disease. That's really interesting because it implies our body is intelligent. We have this innate ability to fight cancer cells and the body tries to boost this by increasing the number of receptors on the cancer cells. Unfortunately, most people are deficient in endocannabinoids or natural cannabinoids. The great thing is that CBD is a perfect supplement.

This study then looked at what happened when these receptors were treated with cannabinoids. The conclusion: "We proved that these treatments produced a cell growth inhibitory effect on all the different prostate cancer cultures."

This means that the treatment stopped or slowed the growth of cancer cells. What's most interesting is that researchers used the word "all," and that's a word that you don't often

---

63 Orellana-Serradell O, Poblete CE, Sanchez C, Castellón EA, Gallegos I, Huidobro C, Llanos MN, Contreras HR., "Proapoptotic effect of endocannabinoids in prostate cancer cells," *Oncology Reports,* 2015 Apr,33(4): 1599-608 EPUB 2015 Jan 21.

see in medical research. They also mention that this effect was demonstrated to be dose dependent.

They go on to say that treatment with endocannabinoids resulted in an increase in a percentage of apoptotic cells (the pre-programmed cell death of cancer cells) and there was a reduction in cancer cells. They believe this was caused by the activation of this apoptotic (cell death) pathway.

"Based on these results, we suggest that endocannabinoids may be a beneficial option for the treatment of prostate cancer that has become nonresponsive to common thera-pies," the study concluded.

Like so many of the studies cited in this book, the research-ers suggest that we could try this natural remedy if other, traditional treatment options don't work. That sounds backward to me. If I was a man with prostate cancer, I might want to try this first, especially when some of the more extreme methods being discussed involve possible castration.

CBD & BREAST CANCER

Now, let's look at a female-specific form of cancer. A 2011 study published in *Molecular Cancer Therapeutics*[64] looked at CBD and how it causes cell death by using the body's

64 Shrivastava A, Kuzontkoski PM, Groopman JE, Prasad A., "Cannabidiol induces programed cell death in breast cancer cells by coordinating the crosstalk between apoptosis and autophagy," *Molecular Cancer Therapeutics*, 2011 Jul; 10(7): 1161-72 EPUB 2011 May 12.

pre-programmed pathway for apoptosis (pre-programmed cell death) and autophagy (which is a related mechanism where your body destroys cells).

Your body destroying cells may sound like a bad thing, but it's always renewing itself, and part of that renewal is more than just making new cells. Let's use bone cells as an example. For your bones to stay healthy, you have osteoblasts, and the osteoblast makes new bone. You also have osteoclasts, and they destroy old bone so you can build new strong bone. Your normal physiology depends on this constant process of destroying old cells and forming new cells. One of the problems with precancerous cells is if your body doesn't naturally detect these cells as it is supposed to, the cells can become cancerous.

You may not realize that all of us have precancerous cells or maybe even cancer cells in our bodies, but our immune system continually detects and destroys them.

In both the laboratory and in the human body, CBD has been shown to fight tumor cells. How? It appears that CBD activates a number of pathways that enhance the ability of crosstalk (or communication) between apoptosis and autophagy. One of the mechanism's studies also found was that CBD tended to destroy the mitochondria (or energy producers) of breast cancer cells, ultimately leading to the death of those cells.

"Our study revealed an intricate interplay between apoptosis and autophagy in CBD-treated breast cancer cells and highlighted the value of continued investigation into the potential use of CBD as an antineoplastic (anticancer) agent," researchers reported.

ONE OF THE DEADLIEST FORMS OF CANCER

All cancer is terrible but one of the worst diagnoses you can receive is that of pancreatic cancer, an extremely malignant form of cancer.

A 2006 study[65] published in *Cancer Research* found an increased number of cannabinoid receptors in pancreatic tumor cell lines and tumor biopsies—much higher than the cannabinoid receptors found in normal pancreatic tissue. They also found that administration of cannabinoids induced the same preprogramed cell death or apoptosis of cancer cells that other researchers found in other types of cancer.

They go on to state that cannabinoids also reduced the growth of tumor cells in two animal models of pancreatic cancer and, in addition, the cannabinoid treatment inhibited the spread of pancreatic tumor cells. Moreover, cells were killed in the pancreatic tumor but not in the healthy tissue. This is important because conventional treatment kills both cancer and healthy cells, which is unfortunately why many people die from the effects of treatment and not the cancer itself.

65 Carracedo A, Gironella M, Lorente M, Garcia S, Guzmán M, Velasco G, Iovanna JL., "Cannabinoids induce apoptosis of pancreatic tumor cells via endoplasmic reticulum stress-related genes," *Cancer Research*, 2006 Jul 1;66(13):6748-55.

"Results presented here show that cannabinoids lead to apoptosis of pancreatic tumor cells," the study concludes. "These findings may contribute to [setting] the basis for a new therapeutic approach for the treatment of pancreatic cancer."

MELANOMA

Melanoma causes the most skin cancer-related deaths worldwide, and protection and early detection are often the only effective measures against it. But that doesn't mean CBD can't have an impact.

The authors of a December 2006 study published in the *Federation of American Societies for Experimental Biology* (FASEB) *Journal*[66] examined new therapeutic strategies for managing this devastating disease with cannabinoids.

It should come as no surprise that their findings echoed the results of other studies. In this case, there was an increase in CB1 and CB2 cannabinoid receptors in human melanoma and also in vitro (studied outside of the body) melanoma cell lines. They found that activating these receptors slowed the growth of new blood vessels. It also decreased the growth of melanoma cells and increased pre-programmed death of melanoma cells in mice.

---

66 Blázquez C, Carracedo A, Barrado L, Real PJ, Fernández-Luna JL, Velasco G, Malumbres M, Guzmán M., "Cannabinoid receptors as novel targets for the treatment of melanoma," *FASEB Journal*, 2006 Dec;20(14):2633-5 EPUB 2006 Oct 25.

As previous studies have shown, researchers also found that only melanoma cancer cells were affected, not healthy cells.

"These findings may contribute to the design of new chemotherapeutic strategies for the management of melanoma," the study concluded.

THE GOLD STANDARD

The proof of all proofs in research is replication—in other words, if you get the same results in controlled conditions over and over again. If you see study after study after study with the same findings, the accumulation of evidence appears to be promising. That is referred to as the gold standard in scientific research, and scientific research to date strongly suggests that someone with cancer might benefit from using CBD.

CBD SAVED MY LIFE

Consider Brittany Brown's experience with CBD and cancer:

"In 2015, I was diagnosed with a benign pituitary adenoma.

"It caused syncopal episodes (loss of consciousness), migraines, slurred speech, severe weight loss, inability to walk, and more. I tried an experimental drug therapy and it put my cancer into remission for a couple years, but it came with significant side effects that included migraines, bloody noses, and vision problems. Because of the drug, I was able to walk again and interact with my daughter, but the tumor was still there.

"Fast forward two years later. After giving birth to my second daughter, my side effects became more severe and included insomnia as well. I was out of options. My neurologist was recommending brain surgery that could potentially leave me in a vegetative state or even kill me. I was told to get my affairs in order and make a will for my two daughters in case I didn't survive the surgery. The grim news was extremely stressful.

"It was at this point when I was introduced to full-spectrum hemp oil CBD. I had nothing to lose so I decided to try it. Seven weeks later, I went in for another brain MRI to map out the size of the tumor as part of the final planning for the surgery. During my follow-up visit the following week, the neurologist walked into the exam room with a big smile and a dumbfounded look on her face. She told me that my brain tumor was completely gone. Not only was there no longer need for surgery, I didn't need to be on medication. I am so thankful for the full-spectrum hemp oil CBD. It literally saved my life!"

CHAPTER SIXTEEN

THE FUTURE OF CBD

The Egyptians recorded symptoms of scurvy as early as 1515 BC, but ancient Greek physician Hippocrates was the first to have documented scurvy as a disease. As early as the thirteenth century, it was known that scurvy was a disease that could be cured by the vitamin C found in common citrus fruits like lemons, limes, and oranges. However, it was not until more than 200 years later that physician, James Lind, scientifically demonstrated scurvy could be treated by supplementing the diet with citrus fruits.

Even with this discovery, more than two million sailors died of scurvy from 1500 to 1800, and scurvy killed more British sailors in the eighteenth century than enemy action. George Anson lost 1,300 of his 2,000 sailors within the first 10 months of a four-year voyage in 1740. At the time, sailors and naval surgeons were well aware that citrus fruits could cure scurvy but classically trained physicians in charge of the medical establishment dismissed the evidence as purely anecdotal. Only in the nineteenth century was it finally accepted that scurvy was a nutritional deficiency best treated by consumption of fresh fruits, particularly fresh citrus fruits and fresh meats. And even then, there were reports of sailors who died from scurvy in the twentieth century.

Scurvy was a disease with a natural treatment. It had been proven over and over again, yet it took more than 300 years and millions of lives before it was properly acknowledged by the medical community. We may live in a more advanced time today but this is an excellent example of how the medical system works and how natural and effective remedies can be overlooked. Things can be extremely slow to change.

The history of scurvy is a good parallel to what we're seeing with a product like CBD. It starts with the way we look at disease. We're not used to the idea of there being one natural supplement or plant that can have such a massive effect on so many different aspects of health. We're so used to looking at pharmaceutical drugs to treat various conditions that we quickly overlook or dismiss products derived from natural foods and plants. The good news is that things are starting to change, and we're experiencing growth in the awareness and availability of a supplement like CBD[67, 68].

In 2018, as I write this book, the Farm Bill is poised to help hemp become a popular commodity and huge cash crop for American farmers by taking it off the list of controlled substances, which it should never have been on in the first place. This is no small feat when considering what

67 Catherine Price, "The Age of Scurvy," *Distillations Magazine from The Science History Institute*, Summer 2017.
68 "The History of Scurvy and Vitamin C," Kenneth J. Carpenter, ed. *Cambridge: Cambridge University Press*, 1986.

the grassroots natural supplement movement is fighting against—for example, the pharmaceutical, hospital, and healthcare industry—in its effort to make hemp and CBD more readily available.

A growing number of medical physicians also are becoming more aware of the benefits of CBD and are open to its use. I would still say that those physicians are in the minority, but I personally know of five physicians in my area who recommend CBD oil to their patients. One of them told me he loves CBD for his patients because it is so safe to use compared to prescription medications.

Word is beginning to spread. I see it in my own clinic. The product took off once we started selling it and hasn't slowed down. We've even had trouble keeping it in stock.

One of the reasons why CBD is such an amazing natural product is because it can help with so many different conditions. This book was organized so each chapter outlined its benefits for specific conditions but when you combine them, it is quite amazing to see that one substance can help with so many things. That is the major difference between a holistic approach to health versus a conventional approach.

While pharmaceutical drugs overpower the body to change the way it works, CBD works with your entire body to allow it to function better. Our bodies have become deficient in cannabinoids, and when we resupply them with CBD, we get them working the way they are intended.

The stage is set for the hemp and CBD industry to explode,

but many people still don't understand the life changing and varied benefits. That is part of my reason for writing this book. In addition to filling society's need for a natural, safe treatment, arguably the most profound benefit of CBD is as a daily supplement to maintain good health. It's always better to prevent health issues before they even occur.

In the words of Dr. David Allen, a retired cardiac surgeon and cannabinoid research scientist at the International Cannabinoid Research Society (ICRS), **"The discovery of the endocannabinoid system is the single most important medical, scientific discovery ever and will save more lives than the discovery and application of sterile surgical technique."**[69]

CAN I GIVE IT TO MY PETS?

Our family's little 15-pound dog is terrified of thunderstorms. In the middle of the night, she'll crawl up to the top of our bed, wake us up, and start to pant. But when I take one drop of CBD and rub it into her gums with my finger, her frightened behavior completely disappears. It's almost like the thunderstorm isn't happening at all.

There is science to back up the use of CBD in pets. In July 2018, *Frontiers of Veterinary Science*[70] published a study that

---

69 https://www.youtube.com/watch?v=LCs4B-oXOdk.
70 Gamble, Lauri-Jo., Boesch, Jordyn M., Frye, Christopher W., Schwark, Wayne S., Mann, Sabine., Wolfe, Lisa., Brown, Holly., Berthelsen, Erin S., Wakshlag, Joseph, J., "Pharmacokinetics, Safety and Clinical Efficacy of Cannabidiol Treatment in Osteoarthritic Dogs," *Frontiers in Veterinary Science,* July 23, 2018.

showed CBD helped to decrease pain in osteoarthritic dogs with no reported side effects. The benefits appear to be very similar to CBD use in humans, and the recommended dose when administering CBD to your dog is one drop per 10 pounds of body weight.

I have heard multiple stories from friends about CBD helping pets. One friend of mine gives CBD to her 17-year-old Labrador with arthritis. She reports that the elderly dog moves much better and seems to be happier. Another friend reported that her large dog would become uncontrollably wild and eat furniture whenever her daughter (who used to own the dog) left the house. She discovered that CBD stopped this behavior.

A PERSONAL NOTE FROM THE AUTHOR

The next step is at www.CBDdrmark.com.

*"The only thing worse than being blind
is having sight and no vision."*

—*Helen Keller*

I hope that my book has given you a vision of what is possible. What might be possible for you personally, or maybe what might be possible for a loved one. Maybe you see the bigger and very real vision of changing your community or taking it beyond your local community to change the world.

I hope you are convinced and you are ready to act. To that, I say, *"You have sight and vision, and together we can change the world."*

The next step is at www.CBDdrmark.com where you can find extensive information about what I believe are the best CBD products on the market as well as ground floor business opportunities in this dramatically growing industry. You'll also find a link to purchase products for shipment directly to you or your loved one's home. Finally, I will be using the www.CBDdrmark.com website to share updated hemp and CBD product and research information as it becomes available.

Remember, the best way to eat an elephant is one bite at a time, and the key to success is often just getting started!

Wishing you health and happiness,

Dr. Mark Lindholm
Chiropractor

DR. MARK A. LINDHOLM

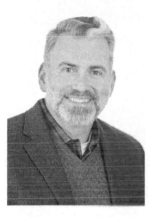

Dr. Mark A. Lindholm has been a chiropractor for over 25 years, specializing in the care of pregnant women, infants, and families. Dr. Lindholm also has extensive experience in the clinical application of nutritional, physical, and lifestyle approaches for optimal health and longevity. He is a frequent lecturer especially on the topics of the clinical applications and financial opportunities of CBD and the Endocannabinoid System. Dr. Lindholm owns and operates the Natural Health Family Chiropractic clinic in Elkhart, Indiana.